Clinical Audit in Primary Care

DEMONSTRATING QUALITY AND OUTCOMES

Ruth Chambers

and

Gill Wakley

Radcliffe Publishing
Oxford ● Seattle

Radcliffe Publishing Ltd
18 Marcham Road
Abingdon
Oxon OX14 1AA
United Kingdom

www.radcliffe-oxford.com
Electronic catalogue and worldwide online ordering facility.

_____

British Library Cataloguing in Publication Data

A catalogue record for this book is available from the British Library.

ISBN 1 85775 709 2

Typeset by Advance Typesetting Ltd, Oxford
Printed and bound by TJ International Ltd, Padstow, Cornwall

Contents

Preface

This book will help you to develop your expertise in clinical audit and collect evidence of your practice. Clinical audit should be an integral part of clinical practice. It can be a powerful tool for positive change, resulting in improved practice and outcomes for patients. Although clinical audit has been promoted and encouraged in the NHS for the last ten years, it is still not practised in a systematic way. Variations in practice between practitioners, or between different practices, may go unnoticed and unchecked if health professionals and managers do not have the knowledge or skills to practise clinical audit, nor the motivation to review their performance in a systematic way.

The umbrella term *clinical audit* includes all the non-clinical components of audit too. You cannot deliver good quality care in a clinical area without looking at access to and availability of care, how good the communication is between staff and with patients, the evidence for your clinical protocols and so on. Everyone in the practice team plays their part. They only operate effectively if they are working in a well connected way within the wider team across primary care and with others in the hospital or community.

This book will help you as a doctor, nurse, allied health professional, manager or other member of the general practice team to undertake clinical audit of any part of your daily practice, but especially in respect of chronic disease management. Clinical audit is key to the way that anyone working in primary care demonstrates that they are playing their part in providing a good service in relation to their role and responsibilities. Health visitors, physiotherapists, podiatrists, pharmacists and others attached to practices will find the information and worked examples in this book useful too.

Most practitioners and managers have patchy knowledge of and skills relating to the various methods of clinical audit and how to act on audit results. Increasing your expertise in clinical audit will help you to gather evidence of your performance and practice. You can use this evidence for improving your clinical or service provision and for the documentation for your appraisal, revalidation or re-registration of your professional qualifications.

Clinical audit helps you to review the way your practice organisation works as a whole – and make improvements. It will not only help you to improve the quality of care you provide but also increase your practice income by boosting reward points from the Quality and Outcomes Framework of the General Medical Services (GMS) contract. Primary care organisations[1] can use clinical audit to demonstrate what standards of care they provide; and how seamless their provision of clinical care is across the boundaries of primary and secondary care, or health and social care or with the voluntary sector.

Ruth and Gill, the authors, work at the 'coalface' of primary care as health professionals and in NHS management. Their positive approach to clinical audit will show you how easy it can be to plan and carry out audit, based on the many useful templates of common conditions included here. These focus on audit from the perspectives of individual members in the primary care team and as a general practice organisation.

Ruth Chambers
Gill Wakley
March 2005

We use the term primary care organisation (PCO) to include primary care trust (PCT) in England; local health group (LHG) in Wales; Health and Social Service Board (HSSB) in Northern Ireland; and the equivalent Local Health Care Co-operative (LHCC) in Scotland.

About the authors

Ruth Chambers has been a general practitioner (GP) for more than 20 years and is currently the head of the Stoke-on-Trent Teaching Primary Care Trust programme and clinical dean at Staffordshire University. Ruth has worked with the Royal College of General Practitioners to produce tools to enable GPs to gather evidence about their learning and standards of practice while striving to be excellent GPs. Ruth has co-authored several series of books with Gill, designed to help readers draw up their own personal development plans or workplace learning plans around key clinical topics, and demonstrate their competence.

Ruth has served as the Chairman of Staffordshire Medical Audit Advisory Group and been a GP trainer. She has scrutinised clinical governance in primary care trusts as a reviewer for the Commission for Health Improvement. Ruth has initiated and run all types of educational initiatives and activities.

Gill Wakley started in general practice in 1966, but transferred to community medicine shortly afterwards and then into public health. A desire for increased contact with patients caused a move back into general practice, together with community gynaecology. She has been combining the two, in varying amounts, ever since.

Throughout she has been heavily involved in learning and teaching. She was in a training general practice, became an instructing doctor and a regional assessor in family planning, and is a visiting professor at Staffordshire University. Like Ruth, she has run all types of educational initiatives and activities from individual mentoring and instruction, to small group work, plenary lectures, distance learning programmes, workshops, and courses for a wide range of health professionals and lay people.

Part 1

The infrastructure of audit

1

Introduction to clinical audit

Getting started with clinical audit

Audit is a technique used to maintain and improve the quality of care and services provided by an individual or by a practice. It is the method used by 'health professionals to assess, evaluate, and improve the care of patients in a systematic way, to enhance their health and quality of life'.[1] Clinical audit is central to clinical governance because:

- you can use it to review the quality of care you provide for patients with common conditions like asthma or diabetes, on an everyday basis
- it builds on the way that health professionals and others working in the NHS have traditionally reviewed case notes as part of quality improvement
- it provides a systematic approach to reviewing the quality of care and services
- it supplies reliable information to highlight the need for improvements
- it provides an impetus to upgrade the quality of care you provide.

Clinical audit is a quality improvement process that seeks to improve patient care and outcomes through systematic review of care against explicit criteria and the implementation of change. Aspects of the structure, processes and outcomes of care are selected and systematically evaluated against explicit criteria. Where indicated, changes are implemented at an individual team or service level and further monitoring is used to confirm improvement in healthcare delivery.[2]

The steps of the audit cycle represented in Figure 1.1 are:

- prioritise and select the topic of your audit, working with others in your team or practice
- set objectives: relating to the reason(s) why the audit is being carried out
- review the literature for that topic and agree the criteria and standards that you think are reasonable
- design the way in which you will do the audit
- collect the data and look at them
- feed back the findings; meet with colleagues or your team to discuss the findings and determine the reasons for the results
- make a timetabled action plan to implement any changes that are needed
- review your standards – should you keep the standards you previously set, are they unrealistic or not challenging enough?
- re-audit – creating successive audit cycles.

Designing your clinical audit

The more time you spend planning and designing the clinical audit, the more likely it is that you can move easily through these various steps of the audit cycle and obtain useful information that everyone owns and agrees to act on. Write down your protocol and share the agreed version so that everyone can see the part they play.

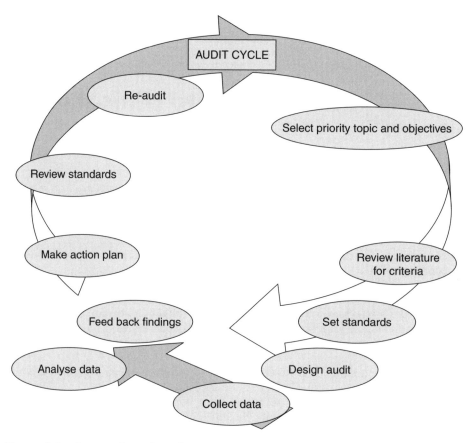

Figure 1.1: Steps in the audit cycle

Who will be involved?

Include those members of the practice team who are directly involved in the task being audited and those who will be collecting the data. Decide who is writing the audit protocol and who will search for evidence to enable you to set standards and criteria. Include in the team those who need to agree solutions or find resources if the audit shows that change is necessary. Appoint a lead if there is no-one in this role already. Link to others relevant to the audit who work in different settings: the local hospital, primary care organisation (PCO), community clinic, social services, etc.

Set simple, measurable, achievable, realistic and timely (SMART) objectives

You should be clear about the reason(s) for doing the audit, and the objective you set should link to that – to define the extent of potential risk areas, for example. The objectives should be relevant and understandable to everyone taking part. Keep in mind that the end result is making improvements to patient care. The quality and nature of the end points of your audit should relate to the objective(s) you set for the audit. You need to have some idea of your endpoint when you set the objective(s). The audit will be most worthwhile if your objective is about:

- assessing whether or not standards are being met
- determining whether standards are improving
- monitoring the level of compliance or concordance with treatment or advice
- improving clinical effectiveness
- changing inadequate current practice.

Box 1.1: Example of objectives of an audit of local services, e.g. management of suspected myocardial infarction

Main objective: to audit the extent to which the following criteria were met and to identify reasons for failure to implement the policy for the management of suspected heart attack:

- the proportion of patients who receive thrombolytic therapy within six hours of the onset of chest pain and within 30 minutes of arrival at hospital
- the length of time patients wait from the onset of symptoms before calling emergency services
- the response time of emergency medical services
- whether aspirin is administered, by whom, and when.

Set criteria

These are items by which you will appraise the indicators of the level of care. The level of performance in your audit results will describe the extent to which these criteria are met. Criteria are explicit statements that define what is being measured; they represent elements of care that can be measured objectively.[2]

Set standards

Standards are indicators of the level of care that you want to achieve. They may be those that you have agreed as a practice team, are promoted by others such as in the Quality and Outcomes Framework,[3] or in other published literature, such as systematic reviews or national clinical guidelines.

Data collection

Decide what information you wish to collect and how to collect it in a reliable way, minimising bias as far as possible. You may need to pilot the collection of data to see how that works out, and solve any problems that arise. Decide if the data collection is retrospective, concurrent or prospective. The data collected must be valid and accurate. The data should be readily available on your computer system or from patient surveys. You will not have time or resources to track down hard-to-locate information.

Define the sample

See page 23 for how you might select your sample of who will be included and excluded from the audit. The number in your sample and the trouble you take to get a representative sample will depend on the accuracy or degree of confidence you need to have in the findings, and the extent to which you are limited by time, funds, staff skills etc.

Data analysis

Decide who will look at the data, how the analysis will be done and how the interpretations will be made.

Feed back the findings

Feedback should be to the people involved in the audit and anyone who will need to make changes. You might be feeding back findings further afield – in your appraisal or in your revalidation or re-registration portfolio, or to the PCO as part of the Quality and Outcomes Framework.

Draw up the action plan

The action plan needs to be timetabled and specific about who does what, how and when – and realistic. The need for any extra resources should be predicted and how they will be identified included in the action plan. If the actions or changes mean new responsibilities for staff, then you need to anticipate their training requirements and organise that training in work or paid time. *See* Chapter 4 for how you might facilitate the changes necessary.

Convene an implementation group

Everyone concerned in the action plan will need to discuss progress with someone taking the lead. If it is a complex audit or crosses more than one health setting, you will probably need an occasional group meeting to oversee progress and agree on re-auditing.

Re-audit

You will want to re-audit if your initial audit showed gaps in the care you are providing and you have made changes as a consequence, to see if you are now meeting, or approaching, the criteria and standards you have set.

Angle what clinical audit you do on:

- a clear patient focus
- greater multiprofessional working
- crossing primary, secondary and continuing or social care boundaries
- close links with education and professional development
- effectiveness – clinical effectiveness, cost-effectiveness, variations in practice, outcomes.

Selecting the topic for audit

You have little enough time to get your core work done in the NHS and you do not have time to waste on doing clinical audit unnecessarily. There must be obvious potential benefits for the audit to be worthwhile to repay the time, costs and effort invested. These benefits include improving the way you deliver care or manage services, or making changes to benefit:

- patients
- your professional practice or personal development
- colleagues
- the practice team
- the practice organisation as a whole
- the PCO or the NHS in general.

Box 1.2:   Categories justifying selecting a clinical audit topic as a priority

An audit topic should concern an area that has at least one of the following characteristics:

- high risk
- high volume
- causes concern
- high cost

The topic or focus of the audit has to be important as in Box 1.2 – to you, your patients, your practice or the NHS in general, or central to local or national initiatives. If the audit is about a clinical condition, then it should concern a common problem, or be related to an aspect of practice with potentially serious consequences if there is underperformance. If it is about practice systems then choose to audit an issue where the audit exercise should help you to work more effectively or efficiently. There must be the potential to make improvements through the audit. There is no point in demonstrating that additional resources are needed to improve some process if there is no chance at all of gaining those additional resources, however hard you try.

The categories that an audit normally falls into include:

- assessing the frequency or volume of a service
- risks associated with aspects of providing care or a service
- problems associated with delivering care or a service
- effectiveness of aspect(s) of the delivery of care or a service
- cost of aspect(s) of delivering care or a service.

Consider if the problem underpinning a topic you are about to select is amenable to change. If not, is there any point in selecting it and carrying out the audit unless that is part of a business case to justify investing resources?

Structure, process and outcome

Performance is often broken down into the three aspects of structure (what you need), process (what you do) and outcome of care (what you expect), an approach recommended by Donabedian.[4] You may choose to focus on any of these three components, or your audit might flow from one to another to include all three aspects in your design.

- *Structural audits* might concern you undertaking audit in relation to what resources you have got, such as diagnostic equipment, premises, access to support services, skills, staffing etc.
- *Process audits* focus on what was done to a patient or how the team operates, for instance how clinical protocols and guidelines work in practice, waiting times, patient recall for investigations, treatment, record keeping, communication etc.
- *Auditing outcomes* relates to the impact of healthcare or services on the patient: improvements, adverse events. You might audit endpoints of providing care such as the effectiveness of care or services on patients' health, patient satisfaction or convenience.

Using audit to monitor services

You could use audit to examine the standards of care or services you provide for any practice-based activities. Make it easy to undertake regular audit by getting into the habit of storing information on a computer in a way that is well coded, accurate and retrievable. Once the parameters for a computerised audit are set up, you can repeat the audit cycle to determine the impact of any changes you make after the initial audit. Be critical of the results, however. Just because you can count something, does not mean that the results are significant in their own right. You need to consider the results in the context from which they were obtained. If the results do not agree with what your common sense tells you is likely to be right, look at how you obtained the data. See if there are significant errors and omissions or biases in the way you organised the sampling, from which you can learn.

Practice-based systems and procedures require regular monitoring for good patient care and the smooth running of the practice organisation. You might monitor:

- systems for the purchase, servicing and maintenance of equipment. Make sure that the people who are responsible for checking equipment (such as the sterilising equipment in your treatment room) have deputies who know their role in case of staff absence or sickness
- staff health – for example, check that you have procedures for ensuring that immunisation against tetanus, rubella and hepatitis is checked before employment, and at recommended intervals thereafter
- confidentiality – to make sure that newly appointed or temporary staff are aware of the rules concerning patient confidentiality, and that breaches of confidentiality do not occur
- safety and maintenance of the premises – that they are clean and present no hazards to staff or patients. You might draw up a list of the statutory and mandatory training required by different practice staff groups, and audit that their training is up to date and that they are complying with health and safety legislation
- that systems and procedures for patient referrals – writing and sending letters and reports, notification of results of investigations to patients, etc are working. You could check that you are copying personal letters to patients according to your agreed practice approach
- waiting times – to see a health professional from the time of the patient request to attending an appointment in your practice, or in relation to time from referrals

being sent from the practice to request outpatient appointments or hospital admissions or investigation dates.

If you wish to extend your audit outside your immediate workplace where you have responsibility, involve colleagues there in the planning and process of the audit. For example, you might want to include services provided in secondary care or in a community department such as physiotherapy.

Setting criteria

The criteria describe the specific items of healthcare or services that you will measure as part of the audit focusing on structure, process or outcome (*see* page 8). For example, a criterion for diabetes is 'patients with diabetes (on your practice list) should have a record of HbA_{1c} or equivalent in the previous 12 months'. Or a criterion for hypertension is 'patients with hypertension (on your practice list) should have a maximum blood pressure (measured in the last 9 months) of 150/90 mmHg or less'.

Compare your performance against external criteria

Look carefully at the evidence for choosing criteria. Often the evidence for what is done is poor or does not exist. You may choose criteria for which there is agreement about 'best practice' from several sources.

Good Medical Practice for General Practitioners describes 'excellent' and 'unacceptable' performance.[5] This approach and most of the criteria and standards in the document can be generalised to all health professionals and managers, whatever their disciplines. An excellent practitioner meets the excellent criteria all or nearly all of the time; a good practitioner meets the excellent practitioner criteria most of the time; and a poor practitioner consistently or frequently provides care in the unacceptable criteria categories. The *Code of Professional Conduct* from the Nursing and Midwifery Council has similar criteria.[6]

You could compare your performance against criteria you select for any of the following components of your everyday work:

- clinical practice
- record keeping
- access and availability
- emergency treatments
- out-of-hours care
- keeping up to date
- providing information to patients and colleagues
- professional–patient relationships
- avoiding discrimination and prejudice
- teamwork
- referring patients
- professional ethics
- best practice in research
- effective use of resources
- conflicts of interest
- handling mistakes or complaints.

Setting standards

Standards may be relative, that is referenced to norms so that you are comparing your standards with those of other people, or absolute, that is referenced to criteria. The standard describes the level of care to be achieved for any particular criterion.[1] Some standards for knowledge, skills and attitudes are included in *Good Medical Practice for General Practitioners* and the *Code of Professional Conduct* (*see* above).[5,6] Some standards can be derived from those set out in the General Medical Services (GMS) contract,[3] which were in turn derived from a mixture of best practice sources.[3,7–9] For instance, a standard for diabetes is '90% of patients with diabetes (on your practice list) should have a record of HbA_{1c} or equivalent in the previous 15 months'. Or the standard for hypertension is '70% of patients with hypertension (on your practice list) should have a maximum blood pressure (measured in the last 9 months) of 150/90 mmHg or less'.[3]

Box 1.3: Standards should be:

- realistic
- measurable
- achievable
- agreed

You might adopt more challenging criteria or standards by being more specific. If you revised the criterion for diabetes given above to: 'patients with diabetes (on your practice list) should have an HbA_{1c} of 7.4% or below in the last 15 months', you might have more difficulty achieving these levels. Then you might revise your standard too as the criterion is so challenging. Perhaps you would lower the percentage to expect that only 50% of patients meet that criterion, rather than the 90% you expected to have had an HbA_{1c} measured in the same time period.

Sometimes special interest groups and specialist associations or societies disagree with the standards set by the National Institute for Clinical Excellence (NICE) or the Scottish Intercollegiate Guidelines Network (SIGN).[7,8] Then you will have to opt for whichever standard or source of evidence is most appropriate for the objective or purpose of your audit – to strive for improvement in standards of care in your practice or provide evidence of your performance for an external body, etc.

You may set minimum, ideal, optimum or arbitrary standards:

- a *minimum* standard is the lowest acceptable standard (this would be 25% for the quality indicators of the Quality and Outcomes Framework for example, before you achieve any reward points)[3]
- an *ideal*, *gold* or *aspirational* standard describes the care or services you would provide under ideal conditions. These ideal conditions might be where you had sufficient resources and patients followed your advice about healthy lifestyles and recommended treatment. In the example given for diabetes, you might then expect 100% of patients to have an HbA_{1c} of 7.4% or less
- an *optimum* standard involves a judgement about what is possible given the available resources and the patient population. The GMS contract indicator for at least 50% of patients with diabetes to have an HbA_{1c} of 7.4% or less to score maximum quality points reflects this balance[3]

- an *arbitrary* standard might be agreed by peers or members of the practice team, for instance. There may be no reliable source of evidence for the nature of your audit or the setting in which you are conducting it. A useful way of setting these standards is to discuss what you or your colleagues would find acceptable as standards. You may find internally set standards like these are more likely to be owned by those setting them, rather than external standards imposed by others, however well meaning. You and your colleagues should then be well motivated to achieve the standards they proposed and agreed.

Working as a practice team, you can compare your own knowledge and usual practice with others and with protocols or guidelines recommended by NICE or any or all of the National Service Frameworks for England or SIGN.[7,8]

Alternatively, you might compare your own practice against a protocol or guideline that is generally accepted at a national or local level. You could audit your practice to find out how often you adhere to such a protocol or guideline, and if you can justify why you deviate from the recommendations where you choose not to follow them.

Make a timetabled action plan for your audit protocol

You know that if you, or whoever is responsible for leading the audit, do not write down a plan as to how to do the audit and put down some timings against actions, it may never get done. So construct a timetable similar to that in Box 1.4 and note down who will do what and by when against the actions.

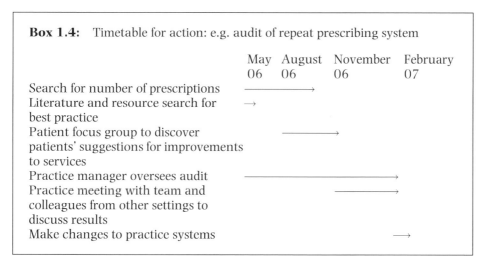

Box 1.4:   Timetable for action: e.g. audit of repeat prescribing system

	May 06	August 06	November 06	February 07
Search for number of prescriptions	⟶			
Literature and resource search for best practice	⟶			
Patient focus group to discover patients' suggestions for improvements to services		⟶		
Practice manager oversees audit	⟶			⟶
Practice meeting with team and colleagues from other settings to discuss results			⟶	
Make changes to practice systems				⟶

Working as a team

Everyone plays their part in the care given to individual patients, from the time they contact the practice for an appointment, to being seen, receiving treatment and investigations and after-care, recording details of their consultation and monitoring any chronic disease. So the design of your audit needs to reflect the way members of your team work together.

Not everyone in the team will need sophisticated knowledge and skills in undertaking clinical audit, but at least one person will need to be able to plan the audit, involve team members in deciding the topic(s) and allocate responsibilities for gathering data, comparing the practice performance with criteria/standards they have agreed are reasonable for their team, planning and making changes.

Your practice team is more likely to function well if it:

- has clear team goals and objectives
- has clear lines of accountability and authority
- has diverse skills and personalities
- has specific individual roles for members
- shares tasks
- regularly communicates within the team – by formal and informal means
- has full participation by team members
- confronts conflict
- monitors team objectives
- gives feedback to individuals
- gives feedback on team performance
- has external recognition of the team
- has two-way external communication between the team and outside world
- offers rewards for the team.[10]

All of these characteristics of good teamworking are pertinent to undertaking clinical audit too. Audit can bind your team together to help each person to realise the part they play in the practice. Really effective teams learn from their errors and problems. Through audit, team members can see what the practice hopes to achieve and how near they are to doing a good job. You might decide to audit the quality of your team working by focusing on any of the components listed above.

Good communication

Good communication is essential for good teamwork and allows audits to be planned and findings shared.[11] You need:

- regular staff meetings – which managers and staff endeavour to attend
- a failsafe system for passing on important messages
- a way to share news so that everyone is promptly notified of changes
- a culture where team members can speak openly without fear of being judged or reprimanded
- opportunities for quieter members of the team to contribute
- to give and receive feedback on how your role in the team is working out
- to praise others for their achievements
- opportunities for team members to point out problems and suggest improvements
- everyone to be part of, and own, the decision making.

Communication is usually poor if a team lacks stability or if single disciplines work in an isolated way. In one study some of the senior doctors were the worst offenders at failing to communicate with others in the team.[12] Power and status issues within a team can interfere with good communication.

Agree a team policy for clinical audit

Agree a written policy about how you will conduct audit in your team or practice. Without it, you may find that you just do audits as the mood takes you, or when there is a deadline pending, such as your annual appraisal. Much better to plan audits in a prioritised and systematic way all year round, spreading the work over the year and across the team in a well ordered way.

Include a statement about how you will identify and agree what issues are important or should be prioritised for audit. State how members of staff can contribute ideas for audit and input their perspectives as to how well the services run. Describe how many audits should be underway at any one time so you do not overload the support staff.

Include an item about preserving confidentiality; individuals should not be identified in any public report shared outside the practice, and those taking part should agree limits on disseminating the findings within and outside the practice team.

Define how often the audit team should meet and how results and subsequent decisions should be communicated to the rest of the team and changes be made. State how findings will be presented to give as accurate and complete a picture of the quality of care and services in the practice as possible.

You will want a section on training and development for all the staff in relation to audit. Everyone should understand what clinical audit means and the benefits to the way the practice runs and patient care, from undertaking audits and acting on the findings. Some staff will need to be able to plan and design audits, and organise data collection. Others will need to analyse the results, and lead on making changes as a result. Hopefully their job descriptions will reflect their roles and responsibilities for audit too.

Share the team policy for audit with other staff attached to the practice or with whom you work closely. Make sure the policy is relevant to them and includes ways that they can link in and share in any of the stages in an audit that the practice runs, as appropriate to their post. Lastly, include a statement about how you will audit the relevance and usefulness of your audit policy!

Feedback of results and action planning in your team

This is a crucial part of your audit. Share the findings with everyone involved so that you can get different perspectives on the issues highlighted by the audit and the type of changes to introduce. The earlier you gain everyone's ownership, the more likely that they will help make changes work.

It is good practice to provide a written report for the team for each audit undertaken detailing the stages of an audit (*see* Figure 1.1) including:

1 why the audit was undertaken
2 what the overall aim and the objectives were
3 the criteria and standards that were used; any definitions
4 the sampling and audit methods employed
5 any procedures used to validate the data
6 the completed action plan
7 changes agreed and made.

Confidentiality

The principle of confidentiality is basic to the practice of healthcare. Patients attend for healthcare in the belief that the information that they supply, or which is found out about them during investigation or treatment, will be kept secret. Health professionals are responsible to patients with whom they are in a professional relationship, for the confidentiality and security of any information obtained. The fundamental principle is that they must not use or disclose any confidential information obtained in the course of their clinical work other than for the clinical care of the patient to whom that information relates.

Exceptions to the above are:

- if the patient consents
- if it is in the patient's own interest that information should be disclosed, but it is either impossible, or
- medically undesirable in the patient's own interest, to seek the patient's consent
- if the law requires (and does not merely permit) the health professional to disclose the information
- if the health professional has an overriding duty to society to disclose the information
- if the health professional agrees that disclosure is necessary to safeguard national security
- if the disclosure is necessary to prevent a serious risk to public health.

Information given to a health professional remains the property of the patient. Generally consent is assumed for the *necessary* sharing of information with other professionals involved with the care of the patient for that episode of care and, where essential, for continuing care. Beyond this, informed consent must be obtained. The development of modern information technology and the increasing amount of multi-disciplinary teamwork in patient care, such as in undertaking clinical audit, make confidentiality difficult to uphold.

The Caldicott principles are nationally agreed guidelines of good practice to safeguard confidentiality when information is being used for non-clinical purposes.[13] These are:

- justify the purpose
- do not use patient-identifiable information unless it is absolutely necessary
- use the minimum necessary patient-identifiable information
- access to patient-identifiable information should be on a strict need-to-know basis
- everyone with access to patient-identifiable information should be aware of his or her responsibilities.

You should tell patients whom you invite to participate in a survey in relation to audit about the standards of confidentiality. You should inform them about the extent to which their identity, contact details and the information they give you is confidential to you, your work team or organisation. Be aware of your responsibilities under the Data Protection Act as to when you need to seek patient consent.[14]

A written confidentiality policy document should be drawn to the attention of all staff in the practice. A named person should be responsible for updating the policy document, monitoring adherence to it and dealing with any potential or actual breaches of confidentiality. Temporary, voluntary or work experience students should all be informed of their obligations to maintain confidentiality. Interpreters should be used wherever possible to avoid the use of friends or relatives. They should be trained in the requirements of confidentiality.

Managers must ensure that paper and computer security is maintained and put into practice systems for monitoring and upgrading security systems. The responsibilities of management, clerical and administrative staff for confidentiality include:

- a clause about confidentiality in contracts of employment
- training in confidentiality for all staff

- a named person with whom any member of staff can discuss difficulties with confidentiality, such as emotional pressure, financial inducement, or lapses by themselves or others
- reporting physical difficulties such as lack of privacy at reception desks or being overheard answering the telephone
- having clear rules about the handling of post marked 'private', 'confidential' or 'personal'
- explaining the reasons for requests for information from patients. Only seeking the minimum of information required for the task
- shredding confidential paper records.

The policy document on confidentiality should contain clear procedures for recording and storing information on paper or on computer. Safeguards against unauthorised access to either must be built in and tested.

Levels of access to data should be clearly stated and passwords to computer records kept confidential (not left on a sticky label on the computer terminal). Terminal security must be arranged so that an unauthorised person is unable to use an unattended terminal to access data. Find out how to organise 'firewall' security against unauthorised access to confidential data. Technology makes sensitive data readily available – not just to those who need to access it.

Blocks and barriers to clinical audit

Your main block to doing clinical audit is probably your inertia or failure to see audit as an integral part of any practice-based activity where the benefits far outweigh the time and effort you take to do it. It is much easier to keep your head down and get on with delivering care than take a little extra time initially to audit how you are doing, consider if you are doing as you intended and to a set standard, make an overall review and change the way you are doing it if your audit findings shows that to be necessary.

The following issues make undertaking audit more difficult or unlikely:[2,15,16]

- failure to participate and negative attitudes to audit: for example, isolation of individual health professionals, even many of those who appear to work in a team
- insufficient involvement of staff from across all the various disciplines
- lack of incentives to undertake audit which is seen as an 'extra' task
- lack of training in audit methodology and evidence-based skills; patchy training of staff carrying out audits
- lack of involvement of patients and service users
- lack of communication between those working in health and social care settings limit applying audit across organisational boundaries, for instance in relation to caring for children
- practitioners overwhelmed with service work perceive that they have too little time for ongoing audit
- lack of resources, especially time
- dissonance between what individuals prefer to audit and what is actually relevant to service needs
- failure to provide a supportive environment for audit; for example, individuals' reluctance to review or monitor their performance, especially if it allows other people to 'inspect' their work
- team members' mental ill-health: depression, stress, burnout – individuals suffering in this way want an 'easy' working life and see audit as yet more hassle

- fear of, and resistance to, change. If you audit some part of your practice, it is likely that it will show you could improve your performance – and that will require a change of some sort
- failure to complete the audit cycle; incomplete implementation of action plans to address the findings of audit and to spread good practice
- cost: of doing audit and implementing improvements.

Try to develop an audit culture in yourself and in your practice – you will soon realise that it will help you as an individual or team to drive up standards, and brings tangible rewards through the Quality and Outcomes Framework.[3]

Involving patients and members of the public

Consumer involvement in audit involves the active involvement of your patients or members of the public in the audit process, rather than engaging them as the 'subjects' of the audit. This involvement might occur in any or all of the processes involved in audit – choosing which topics to audit, planning the way the audit is undertaken, carrying out the audit, interpreting the findings, deciding on changes, and disseminating the results or changes made.

The patient's perspective of the care you deliver or services they experience is crucial for successful audit. Patients can tell you about problems and gaps. Otherwise you may be fooling yourselves that the quality of care and services is acceptable to patients when in reality it is not.[17]

You may need to train a few patients to be able to plan and design audits with you, and analyse and interpret findings. They will need to understand limits on resources and competing priorities if they are to help you plan changes. You will need to be careful about anonymising any data collected and making sure that no patients or professionals can be identified in tables of results when sharing audit findings with patients who are helping you in your audit work.

The difference between audit and research

It has become even more important to distinguish between audit and research since the introduction of research governance management by the NHS. If the bureaucracy of completing application forms for research ethics approval from the local ethics committee or research governance from the local manager, or applying for an honorary contract to do research seems daunting, then NHS staff may be tempted to term their proposed project an *audit* when it is really *research*.

Research determines what constitutes good care and what best practice is. It is concerned with discovering the right thing to do. It is about discovering new knowledge – such as about how well new treatments work.

Clinical audit looks at how well that good care is being practised, or how well services are delivered. It is a way of finding out whether you are doing what you should be doing. It is about determining the extent to which best practice is being applied.

Those undertaking research and clinical audit use similar methods. Both research and audit answer a specific question phrased by an objective(s). They both involve sampling, questionnaire design or other method of collecting data such as patient surveys, scrutinising records, or interviews, and analysis of findings. Data collection in both research and audit can be carried out prospectively, concurrently or retrospectively.

Some of the differences between research and audit appear in Table 1.1.

Table 1.1: Some of the differences between research and audit

Research	Audit
• Creates new knowledge about what does or doesn't work	• Checks if you are following best or agreed standards of practice
• Carried out on a large scale over a prolonged period so that results can be generalised to other populations	• Usually carried out on a relatively small population over a short time span, with the possibility of returning to re-audit later
• Patients may receive a new treatment or other intervention	• Patients never receive a new treatment or other intervention
• The nature and size of the sample population should be scientifically valid	• The sampling is on a smaller scale, sometimes pragmatic and acceptable for the purpose and design of the audit
• Researchers generally publish their results and leave others to act upon them	• Acting on audit findings is the responsibility of the clinical lead or managers involved

There are some areas like patient surveys where it can be difficult to be sure whether they fall within the definition of research or audit. Similarly, staff surveys might be construed as research or auditing a management function. In all cases of uncertainty, you should seek the advice of the chair of your local research ethics committee or the research governance manager.

An audit protocol

Audits come in all shapes and sizes. They may focus on the structure, process or outcome of your service. They could be a snapshot or could follow practice at intervals or continuously – the format and approach depend on the purpose of the audit or your stated objective(s). The following protocol captures all the stages as a checklist for you when designing your audit and making sure it will be worthwhile. If you cannot justify why the audit that you are planning is a priority, scrap the audit you were mapping out and change your focus. Working through each stage of the protocol will force you to consider how you will collect the data and refine your method so that the audit does not become too onerous and unworkable. You will have to think through how you will deal with the data and the outcomes of your audit – so if you do not envisage the findings being useful to you in your practice you have an opportunity to re-angle your audit at the planning stage.

You could use the following audit protocol to help your team or colleagues formulate and check their ideas in preparing an audit. Photocopy the pages so that everyone has a copy to complete.

Checklist to complete to design your audit protocol

1 Choose a topic that is a priority for you or your colleagues or the NHS in general. What is it?

2 What problem are you addressing?

3 How did you choose the topic? Was it (circle all that apply):
- in discussion with other colleagues
- decided on behalf of your work colleagues
- the practice team requested the topic
- a topic in the practice business plan
- a topic in the strategic plan prepared by the primary care organisation (PCO)
- practice manager's recommendation
- patient's or carer's request
- other (write in):

4 Why did you choose this topic? Is it a priority topic?   Yes/No

If yes, is it a priority for (circle all that apply):
- the PCO's strategic plan
- the government
- your trust or PCO
- patients
- your practice team
- certain colleagues
- yourself

- the profession
- National Service Framework (NSF) (which one?)

- National Institute for Clinical Excellence (NICE)
- a previous or recent significant event (organisational, clinical or performance)
- other (write in):

5 Is the topic important?   Yes/No

If yes, is it (circle all that apply):

- high cost
- a common problem
- life threatening
- a need relating to your local population
- a routine check of everyday care or services
- evidence that current care is inadequate
- part of the Quality and Outcomes Framework (QOF)

Why else is it important to audit this topic?

6 What are your objectives? Are they simple, measurable, achievable, realistic and timely?

7 Have you designed your audit protocol in sufficient detail for everyone to know who is doing what, why, when and how?

8 What principles of good practice are included in your audit protocol (circle all that apply)?

- organise multidisciplinary input
- involve colleagues as appropriate
- consider the interfaces of how and where you work with other NHS professionals, the non-health sector and care settings

- incorporate input from patients (e.g. those using your services, carers, the public; at training, planning, monitoring or delivery stages)
- be capable of achieving health gains
- be based on evidence-based practice, policy or management
- if you are a clinician or member of the support staff, incorporate input and commitment from managers to enable action to take place, e.g. protected time for staff involved

9 Who will lead the audit initiative?

10 Who else will be involved?

11 What resources do you need to undertake the audit? Remember training, materials, facilities, skills, people, time.

12 What criteria have you selected and why?

13 What standards have you selected and from where did they originate?

14 What data or information will you gather as a baseline?

15 When will you start? What is the timetable?

16 What system do you have for reviewing the results of the audit exercise and comparing your performance with pre-agreed standards? Who will decide and who will make any necessary changes as a result of the exercise?

17 What changes do you hope to make?

18 Are these changes possible with your current resources and skills? From where will you obtain any additional resources?

19 Are you being realistic in expecting change?

20 How do your findings compare with those of other practices, or across a PCO?

21 What interventions or changes in services or practice will you introduce if your performance does not reach the standards that you have set? What resources will you need for these interventions or changes?

22 What specific outcomes do you expect from introducing the intervention(s) or change(s)?

23 How will you measure outcomes of interventions?

24 How will you demonstrate any improvements or changes from the baseline arising from the intervention(s)?

25 When and how will you re-audit your improved or changed practice or services?

References

1 Irvine D and Irvine S (eds) (1991) *Making Sense of Audit*. Radcliffe Medical Press, Oxford.

2 NHS National Institute for Clinical Excellence, Commission for Health Improvement, Royal College of Nursing and University of Leicester (2002) *Principles for Best Practice in Clinical Audit*. Radcliffe Medical Press, Oxford.

3 General Practitioners Committee/The NHS Confederation (2003) *New GMS Contract. Investing in general practice*. British Medical Association, London.

4 Donabedian A (1966) Evaluating the quality of medical care. *Millebank Memorial Fund Quarterly*. **44**: 166–204.

5 General Practitioners Committee and Royal College of General Practitioners (2002) *Good Medical Practice for General Practitioners*. Royal College of General Practitioners, London.

6 Nursing and Midwifery Council (2002) *Code of Professional Conduct*. Nursing and Midwifery Council, London.

7 www.nice.org.uk

8 www.sign.ac.uk

9 Spooner A (2004) *Quality in the New GP Contract*. Radcliffe Medical Press, Oxford.

10 Hart E and Fletcher J (1999) Learning how to change: a selective analysis of literature and experience of how teams learn and organisations change. *Journal of Interprofessional Care*. **13(1)**: 53–63.

11 Chambers R and Davies M (1999) *What Stress in Primary Care!* Royal College of General Practitioners, London.

12 Miller C, Ross N and Freeman M (1999) *Shared Learning and Clinical Teamwork: new directions in education and multiprofessional practice*. The English National Board for Nursing, Midwifery and Health Visiting, University of Brighton, Sussex.

13 Department of Health (1997) *Report of the Review of Patient-identifiable Information*. In: The Caldicott Committee Report. Department of Health, London.

14 Department of Health (1998) *Data Protection Act 1998. Protection and use of patient information*. Department of Health, London.

15 Healthcare Commission (2004) *State of Healthcare Report*. Healthcare Commission, London.

16 Royal College of Obstetricians and Gynaecologists (2003) *Understanding Audit*. Clinical governance advice No 5. Royal College of Obstetricians and Gynaecologists, London.

17 Chambers R, Drinkwater C and Boath E (2003) *Involving Patients and the Public. How to do it better* (2e). Radcliffe Medical Press, Oxford.

2

Audit methods

Look at your audit objectives and the reason(s) why you are carrying out an audit. Then choose one of the different varieties of audit methods to suit your investigation. You might use audit to:

- set appropriate standards for your future performance
- find out how you are doing compared with others
- find out how you are doing compared with external criteria or standards
- investigate a complaint or significant event
- identify your learning needs, for example about aspects of clinical care
- discover what service developments are needed, for example about access to, or availability of, services.

By now, after graduating from Chapter 1, you know that if the audit shows that you need to make changes, you should make an action plan to implement the changes and then re-audit to ensure that things have improved.

Sampling[1]

You do not have to ask the opinion of every patient registered with your practice to find out patients' views about how your services perform. For example, looking at the availability of appointments, you can get that information by asking a sample of the practice population and looking at the records of appointments bookings. But to get an accurate answer, the sample you select should represent the whole of your practice population. If you were to ask every patient attending a Monday morning surgery how easy it had been to make their appointment, you would only be asking people who had been able to overcome any difficulties in gaining an appointment and could attend surgery during working hours on a Monday. There might still be many people excluded from your enquiry who had not been able to get through on the phone or who had voiced their request in such a way that they had received a prescription or advice instead of an appointment, who had no transport, or who could not attend during working hours on a Monday. Monday morning surgery might not be a good time to do an audit, as there might be different access problems when the surgery has been closed for two days over the weekend, than on other days of the week.

Composing your sampling frame

The *population* is the total group that you are interested in auditing, for example those with severe mental health problems or people in your practice population known to have diabetes. Usually you will have to select a sample of the population of patients for the audit, unless the target population is very small (e.g. users of your services with a very rare condition such as those patients prescribed lithium), or your resources are infinite (which is very unlikely).

In order to select a sample of the population, you will need to produce a *sampling frame*. A sampling frame is a list of members of the population from which the sample is drawn. This can be whatever you choose, for example all patients on a practice disease register, all patients admitted to a ward over a selected interval, or all people with severe mental health problems in one geographical area. However, you may not always have a sampling frame from which to select a sample. For example, you might not be able to identify a sampling frame for illegal drug users, or people caring for relatives with dementia.

As the example in Box 2.1 demonstrates, getting the sampling frame wrong results in sampling errors that can have significant consequences.

Box 2.1:   Example of a sampling error

In 1936, a poll carried out by the *Literary Digest* predicted that Roosevelt would be defeated in the presidential election. Although it was based on a poll of several million people, it was wrong. The reason for this was that the sample was mainly taken from car registration lists and telephone directories. In 1936 many voters did not own a car or a telephone, and those who did were well off compared to the general population. The sampling frame was not representative of the general voting population and was incorrect.

A number of sampling strategies you might use are outlined in Box 2.2. Your choice of sampling strategy will vary depending on the type of audit or patient/staff partici-pation initiative that you plan to carry out, the people you wish to include in your sample and whether or not you have a sampling frame and the resources available to you.

Box 2.2:   Sampling strategies[1] (modified from Blaxter *et al.* 1996)[2]

Probability sampling

- *Simple random sampling* – select a group of patients at random from your practice register or from a particular disease register
- *Systematic sampling* – select every *n*th patient from a practice register
- *Stratified sampling* – sample within patient groups on your practice register
- *Cluster sampling* – survey whole clusters of patients at random

Non-probability sampling

- *Convenience sampling* – sample the most convenient group of patients (or carers) you can find
- *Voluntary sampling* – the sample is made up of patients using your practice who self-select
- *Quota sampling* – convenience sample within patient groups of the practice population
- *Purposive sampling* – hand-picked sample of typical or interesting patients
- *Snowball sampling* – building up a sample through patients or other members of the public who know people with similar conditions

---

Other kinds of sampling

- *Event sampling* – using routine or special events as the basis for sampling
- *Time sampling* – recognising that different parts of the day, week or year may be significant, for certain patients or groups (e.g. people with a chronic disease such as diabetes) and sampling accordingly

---

The sampling technique you use is very important as you are trying to select a sample that can be trusted to represent the whole population to which the question underlying your audit applies. Think of ways to sample that are as little biased as possible, yet do not generate an unrealistic amount of work for you.

Data collection

The type and extent of information you require usually becomes clear as you design the audit. Most data collected is numerical or quantitative, but it can be useful to collect more descriptive or qualitative information to understand complex areas such as the views of service users. Think carefully about the amount of data you want to collect. Generally the fewer the items you include, the more accurately they will be recorded. If you try to look at large numbers of items in one audit, its purpose will lack clarity, and necessary changes will not be easy to identify.

It will usually be obvious whether you record prospective or retrospective data (*see* Table 2.1).

Table 2.1: Prospective or retrospective data

	Retrospective	*Prospective*
Definition	Data recorded from past records	Data collected from this point onwards or from a point in the future
Use	Looking at what has happened in a defined area	If data are not currently available (e.g. when something new is introduced) When past data are poor or incomplete
Advantages	Can be quick to do	Avoids using incomplete or poor data
	Provides a baseline	Permits the design of clear and concise data collection sheet
Disadvantages	Past service users do not benefit	Can be time consuming as you have to wait for sufficient numbers
	Data may be difficult to find or incomplete	

As with all data collection make sure that information is collected in a way that is both valid and reliable:

- *validity* is the degree to which you are measuring what you are supposed to be measuring e.g. waiting time from when the patient was due to be seen, to going into the consulting room, not including the time that he or she checked in half an hour before the time of the appointment
- *reliability* is the degree to which you are consistently measuring what you want to measure, e.g. the same data would be collected by another person, or at a different time. For example, you cannot assume that blood pressure measurements are reliable unless you are sure that sphygmomanometers are regularly calibrated and doctors, nurses and healthcare assistants trained to heed best practice guidance on taking blood pressures.

Using standardised data collection tools increases the validity and reliability of your data collection. A well-tested questionnaire will avoid the pitfalls of poor design leading to unreliable data. If you cannot find a collection tool that has been tested elsewhere, ensure that you pilot yours first to iron out any difficulties.

You can improve the reliability of data collection by training all those who are providing the data in correct methods of data entry. For example, ensure that everyone is using the correct Read codes for chronic diseases as they enter information on the computer.

Types of audit

Case note analysis

You can undertake a retrospective review of a random selection of notes, or carry out a prospective survey of what is done for, or with, consecutive patients with the same condition, e.g. diabetes. The analysis provides insight into your current practice. Set your standards after reference to the literature about best practice in managing that clinical condition. Then compare your performance with those standards or levels of performance.

Looking at the history of the care of an individual patient is the richest material for expanding knowledge and understanding. Use examination and review of cases for whom you have provided care, for professional development and improving care for patients.

Peer review

Compare an area of your practice with how other individual professionals or managers work; or compare aspects of the performance of your practice team as a whole with what others do. An independent body like a local university or an audit resource might compare all practices in one area, for example, within the primary care organisation (PCO). This needs to be well organised so that like is compared with like. Feedback is usually given in a way that protects participants' identities. Only the individual person or practice knows their own identity, the rest being anonymised, perhaps by being given a number. In a well-established group where there is mutual trust and an open learning culture, peer review does not need to be anonymised as far as participants' identities go, and everyone can learn together about making improvements in practice.

So you might decide on a particular audit design with one or more other practitioner or practice, collect the data and compare the results, working together giving feedback on each others' performance.

Criteria-based audit

This compares your clinical practice against specific indicators of performance, guidelines or protocols you derive from national publications or accepted sources such as the Quality and Outcomes Framework (QOF).[3] Following the changes identified as necessary, re-audit should demonstrate improvements in the quality of patient care and more reward points if relevant to the QOF.

External audit

Audit facilitators, prescribing advisers and primary care development managers can supply you with data relating to indicators of your performance that may be useful in carrying out audits. However, all the relevant members of the practice team have to be involved and use the information in an audit capacity to encourage their ownership and commitment to make any necessary changes in practice. Practice visits from external bodies, such as those linked to accreditation for an award organised by the Royal College of General Practitioners (RCGP), or an inspection as a general practitioner (GP) training practice, expose the practice and individual practitioners to external audit.

Direct observation

Collect your data by recording what is observed. Direct observation of consultations or procedures by a person or audio- or videotaping can often be more accurate than written records that were collected for another purpose and only used for audit in an incidental way.

Patients' or staff observations can be collected using a structured enquiry form to give consistency.

Surveys

Patient satisfaction surveys may seem to be relatively easy to organise, but their shortcomings, such as bias in the sample or poor return rates, can outweigh their usefulness. Having set standards, you might carry out a survey as a general indicator of care or for detecting a problem, rather than as an accurate measure of performance. Beware that you do not trespass into the territory of research and require ethics approval for your audit (*see* page 16). Use a validated tool such as the General Practice Assessment Questionnaire (GPAQ) and the Improving Practice Questionnaire (IPQ) which have been accepted as valid measures of patient views.[4,5] Issue these to patients on an annual basis. You can post out the questionnaires or give them out to patients in the surgery. The questionnaires look specifically at access, the quality of the consultation itself and the information given out and the quality of the premises and other parts of the practice that patients have experienced.

The questionnaires are standardised and have been used extensively in British general practice. The GPAQ instrument is free to use, and printed copies can be obtained for a fee. The IPQ instrument is not free but the cost includes printed questionnaires and analysis.

Tracer criteria

Assessing the quality of care of a tracer condition may be used to represent the quality of care of other similar conditions or more complex problems, for example, the extent to which you adhere to pre-agreed clinical protocols, guidelines and care pathways. Tracer criteria should be easily defined and measured. Ensure that they are relevant to the condition being studied. When you come to look at the findings, does being unable to justify deviations from the agreed procedures reveal any learning needs?

Significant event audit

A significant event may be an identified risk, a near miss, or something that actually caused harm. The term significant event audit includes adverse and critical events. A significant event audit is a structured approach to reviewing events that have occurred in your practice. Such events might be in any area of work: prevention, acute care, chronic disease, organisation or management. Significant event auditing should be a positive developmental process.

These days, significant event audit is expected as a norm, so include significant event audits in the evidence of your practice that you have in your appraisal or revalidation portfolios, or the evidence of your practice performance for the Quality and Outcomes Framework. Many practices have set up their own significant event forms so that events can be easily recorded and circulated to the practice team for collection of further data. The practice uses the forms as a basis for discussion to identify what, if any, changes need to be made, by whom and how they will be implemented.

Discuss the completed significant event audit at a meeting of the GPs and nurses, the primary care team or within a special interest group. Determine what lessons can be learned, what areas require further work on your part, how care can be improved, who is responsible for the action plan and by when. Significant event auditing, critical incident analysis and adverse event monitoring all contribute to the risk management and quality enhancement within a practice.

Significant events can give an understanding of the care that individual practitioners or the practice team deliver. While all significant events have the capacity to be identified as areas for improvement, most can also demonstrate good or appropriate care. For example, when a 65-year-old man is diagnosed as having a bronchial carcinoma, this is a 'significant' event. A review of the case notes might demonstrate that 'best' care was delivered – he had been asked about his smoking habits and appropriate advice had been given; he had been diagnosed quickly and referred appropriately. Usually, at least some elements of care are found to be less than perfect; for instance, his cough may not have been investigated early enough, or his smoking habit may not have been addressed.

Adverse events

Some significant events are adverse events. These are events where something clearly has gone wrong, and the practice needs to establish what happened, what was preventable and how to respond. Adverse events might include:

- a patient's complaint
- an allergic reaction to a drug that was already known about
- a request for a home visit taken but the visit not done
- a prescribing error
- an unexpected death
- an unplanned pregnancy
- an avoidable side-effect from prescribed medication
- a violent attack on a member of staff
- an angry outburst in public by you or a work colleague.

The sort of questions you might pose when unravelling the reasons and collecting the data for an adverse event audit are given in Box 2.3.

Box 2.3: A minimum data set for adverse event and near miss reporting

- *What happened?* A description of the events, the severity of actual harm or potential risk, the people and equipment involved
- *Where did it happen?* Location and type of service provided
- *When did it happen?* Date and time
- *How did it happen?* Immediate or approximate causes. Determine the human and other factors most directly associated with the event, and the processes and the systems
- *Why did it happen?* The underlying or root cause(s). Identify risk points. The answer to 'why' might help to redesign service to minimise recurrence of adverse event
- *What action was taken or is proposed?* Immediate and longer term
- *What impact did the event have?* Harm to the patient, organisation, others
- *What factors influenced the impact?* How they acted in minimising or exaggerating the effects

---

Critical incident

A critical incident is an event that may indicate substandard care, but also might have occurred by chance. Any allergic reaction to a drug would be a critical incident, with the investigation aimed at establishing whether it was avoidable. Other critical incidents might be an osteoporotic fracture, a stroke or an unplanned teenage pregnancy – all potentially avoidable and all possibly indicators of deficiencies in healthcare.

Box 2.4:   Example of a significant event audit for you to try

Carry out a significant event audit of two patients with a recent diagnosis of
pelvic inflammatory disease. Establish if any factors emerge that could have
altered the development of the condition. Read up about the risk factors for
pelvic inflammatory disease and consider what procedures might help to
identify patients at risk, and increase the possibility of screening, investigation
and/or early treatment. Present your findings at a meeting for colleagues and
staff to plan changes in their practice or learn from.

Risk management analysis

In every consultation, there is a chance that the process of care might be suboptimal.
Risk management is the process by which you reduce that chance. Efficient administrative systems, a good complaints procedure, decision support, conventional auditing,
error trapping (e.g. double checking of prescriptions) and a positive culture towards
quality are all part of good risk management. Box 2.5 gives ideas for what you can do
as an individual or as a team to practise effective risk management.

Box 2.5:   Promoting effective risk management

What your practice team can do

- Encourage colleagues to actively report patient safety incidents that happen
  (including near misses)
- Participate in reviews, audits and reflective practice activities to share good
  practice and lessons learned

What you can do

- Report patient safety incidents that you encounter
- Report risks and hazards that you notice
- Use reflective practice as part of your continuing professional development
  (CPD) activity and share what you learn with your colleagues

---

Analysis of critical or significant incidents should focus on organisational factors as
well as the performance of particular individuals, as in the example in Box 2.6. The
reason for an adverse event occurring is often outside the control of an individual
practitioner, although they may have contributed to it.

Box 2.6:   Example of an organisational response to a significant event audit

A woman attends her GP's surgery on a Friday evening after the practice nurse
has left and the doctor is out on a visit. She says that she needs to see the nurse,
as she needs the pill urgently. The receptionist gives her an appointment for
Monday morning. On Monday, it is discovered that she actually wanted
emergency contraception and is now outside the 72 hours for oral methods.

She is angry and upset that she now needs to arrange to see a doctor for an intrauterine device to be fitted. A review, run as a significant event audit, of the circumstances prompts some changes. The receptionists learn more about emergency contraception and have some role-play training for dealing with potentially embarrassing situations at the desk. The practice nurses have some extra training and take over more of the emergency contraception provision; their hours are changed slightly so that there is better cover on Friday evenings. No changes to the arrangements for intrauterine device fitting are made, as the number fitted in the practice does not justify it.

Root cause analysis

Root cause analysis (RCA) is promoted by the National Patient Safety Agency (NPSA).[6] It offers a simple framework for gathering and analysing data in a systematic way that works backwards from the incident and builds up a picture of the environment, people and actions involved. The NPSA advocate reporting systems in each practice, PCO and other trusts to provide a core of sound, representative information on which to base your analysis and recommendations. NHS organisations should have (or be developing) a centralised system that gathers data on patient safety incidents. It should cover:

* incidents that have occurred (adverse events or harms)
* incidents that have been prevented (near misses)
* incidents that may happen (risks).

The recommended approach to learning from adverse events and near misses as a practice or PCO is to:[6]

* identify and record reportable adverse events
* report to an overall monitoring body, e.g. the person or group monitoring significant events in the practice or PCO
* analyse the incident, including a root cause analysis, noting any trends
* learn lessons from the analysis, research or other sources of information
* disseminate lessons
* implement change(s) in workplace, at a local or national level as appropriate.

How to do significant event auditing

Identify the group in your practice team with whom you will discuss your cases or events. This group should be as close to you as possible, be signed up to a no-blame culture, and share mutual trust and respect. The culture must be one in which everyone is committed to high-quality care and is willing to improve. It is wise to establish ground rules about confidentiality at an early stage. Discussions within significant event audit meetings and the minutes of the meetings must be treated as confidential.

Agree the type of events that will normally be listed at regular significant event meetings but allow anyone to add any other event. If anyone requests that a particular event is not discussed in open meeting, then that wish should be respected. Box 2.7 describes typical events that might qualify for discussion at significant event audit meetings.

Box 2.7: List of events that might be routinely discussed in significant event audit group meetings

- *Primary prevention*
  - cases of whooping cough, rubella, mumps or measles
  - unplanned pregnancies
- *Diagnostic acumen and delays*
  - new diagnoses of cancer deaths in patients under the age of 75 years
- *Primary/secondary prevention, response to emergencies and rehabilitation*
  - new myocardial infarctions
  - new strokes
  - visits for asthma, diabetes or epilepsy
  - a seizure in patient on anticonvulsant drugs
  - osteoporotic fracture
  - avoidable hospital admission for chronic disease
- *Patient experience of the service*
  - patient suggestions or comments
  - patients' compliments
  - patients' and others' complaints
- *Practice organisation*
  - home visit accepted but not done
  - referral letter not sent
  - medical record or information missing
  - excessive waiting times
- *Risk management*
  - prescribing error
  - lack of regular monitoring of drug, e.g. warfarin

Everyone in the group should record relevant events within the agreed categories, such as those in Box 2.7. The multidisciplinary meeting should reflect and analyse what the triggers, causes and consequences of the event were, and if there is anything individuals or the practice as a whole might do to avoid a similar event happening in future.

Many of the cases can be taken from discharge summaries or patients' letters, or from the practice computer if everyone in the practice team codes diagnoses and encounters, systematically. Before the meeting, someone should draw the reported events together, compile a master list and obtain relevant patient records.

The significant event audit meeting

The notes of the previous meeting should be discussed and checked to see that action has been taken as previously agreed. Each person present should describe one of the significant events they have listed to the rest of the group. The group discusses and prioritises which audits to undertake.

One person records the discussion and agreed actions as listed in Box 2.8. These are typed up with the age and sex of the patient and a computer reference number, but no other patient identifiers.

Box 2.8:   Steps in the analysis of a significant event

- Consider the events to be audited
- Collect data on these events
- Hold a meeting – discuss individual events and some/all of the following aspects:
    - immediate management of the case
    - preventive care opportunities
    - follow-up of the case
    - implications for the family/community
    - interface issues
    - team issues
    - action to be taken/policy decisions to be made
    - follow-up arrangements
- Complete the documentation

Four key outcomes of a significant event discussion

- *Celebration* – how often do you celebrate good care? An example would be if a practice nurse notices an elderly man is 'not himself' when he attends for an influenza immunisation and takes some blood that shows that his anaemia is due to a leukaemia.
- *Immediate change* – where the evidence is clear and the case for change is obvious and agreed. For example, a doctor realises after giving an injection in a patient's home that the vial is out of date, which leads to an agreement to a system of regularly checking drugs in doctors' bags.
- *An audit or investigation is required* – further evidence is required to establish the nature of the problem. For example, a 55-year-old man dies of a myocardial infarction. In discussion, it becomes clear that his brother and father both died young of ischaemic heart disease. How many of your middle-aged men have had their family history recorded? An audit is then arranged to find out.
- *No action* – this is a case of normal general practice where changes have already been made or there is no other action that could be taken to minimise the chance of that significant event happening again.

Who should attend the significant event audit meeting?

It is common for significant event meetings to start off with a few enthusiastic clinicians and then to gradually involve other professionals and staff, as confidence increases. The group may consist of:

- GP(s) and GP registrar(s)
- GP locum – if he or she works at the practice regularly
- practice manager
- practice nurses
- community nurses
- allied health professionals
- senior receptionists
- secretaries.

In time, patients or carers, and all health professionals attached to a practice – counsellors, physiotherapists, dentists, pharmacists – might be invited.

The outcome

Significant event auditing is equally as useful for gathering insights into personal practice for personal development as for improving the practice's organisational care and services. You *could* undertake a significant event audit as a single practitioner. This might be useful if you move between practices as a GP locum. It is likely to be more effective as a practice team or a group of practitioners working together. There will be more opportunity for everyone to be committed to instituting changes in procedures if they have shared the analysis and planned the solution together around real-life examples of patient care. Reviewing individual cases in this way will be a test of the learning culture that you have managed to create in the practice. Everyone can learn from any mistakes or omissions that have been made. An example of a grid that can be used to record your learning needs is given in Table 2.2.

Organising 360° feedback

360° appraisal is a useful way to provide individuals with a varied feedback about their performance or attitudes from their peers, managers, staff members, work colleagues and sometimes patients too. That is, all the people with whom you have contact at work. The tool collects together perceptions from a number of different participants as in Figure 2.1. It is a good way to hear others' personal insights into how you work and behave.

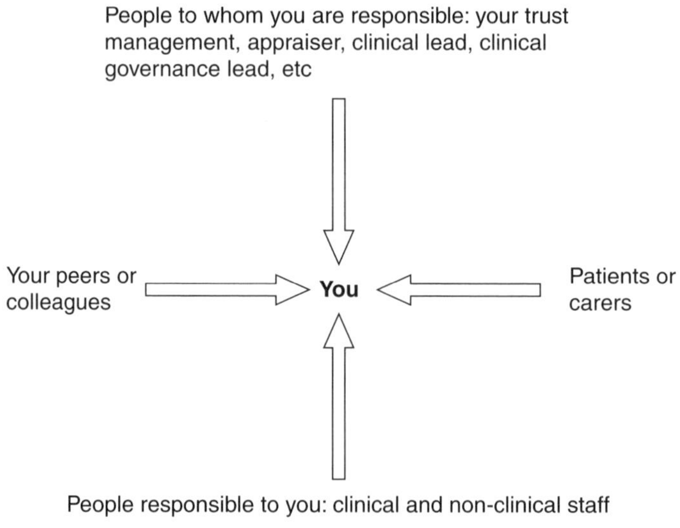

People to whom you are responsible: your trust management, appraiser, clinical lead, clinical governance lead, etc

Your peers or colleagues → **You** ← Patients or carers

People responsible to you: clinical and non-clinical staff

Figure 2.1: 360° feedback

The wider the spread of people giving feedback, the more rounded the picture. Each individual gives a feedback questionnaire to at least five people in each of the groups above. Run the feedback exercise so that it is non-confrontational, non-judgemental, friendly and confidential. It helps to have an independent person to collect and collate

Table 2.2: Recording your learning needs from significant event discussion

Patient reference, sex, age	Event	Learning need	Action

Table 2.2: continued

Patient reference, sex, age	Event	Learning need	Action

the anonymised questionnaires and be ready to discuss the results with individuals who want it. The main disadvantage of this method is that it can sometimes be spoilt by malicious comments against which individuals cannot readily defend themselves if they were anonymous.

If you use this method, look at the feedback and consider:[7]

- what key points have arisen?
- are there any patterns?
- how do you feel about the feedback?
- how does it compare with how you see yourself?
- do you think the feedback is fair?
- does it ring true or are you surprised by the replies?
- what areas will you include in your personal development plan?

The NHS Modernisation Agency's Leadership Centre provides a model for a 360° assessment process. For further information about the tool and how to access it go to the website.[8]

Audit of a service

Just as with clinical audit, you must be sure that spending time reviewing the quality of a particular service is worthwhile. That means it must concern an important aspect of your work that crops up sufficiently frequently to justify the effort spent on audit.

You might audit:

- the range of services provided between practices – specialist services in particular settings; patients' choice of doctor/nurse; approaches to prevention and treatment
- the appropriateness of the services provided – the extent to which your services are geared to meeting local needs
- accessibility of services – where located, opening times
- information – variety of type, options for non-English speakers
- publicity – the extent to which patients are aware of the type and availability of services
- skill mix – staffing levels
- training of staff – whether they are working within their competencies, and there are sufficient opportunities for CPD
- good employer practices for staff – regular appraisal, regard for health of staff at work, good communication with staff at all levels by the practice manager
- whether underlying reasons for any failure to meet standards were identified.

An example of an audit of services appears in Box 2.9.

Box 2.9: Example of an audit on contraceptive services

Is it a priority topic?
There are more than 100 000 terminations in the UK per year, and many sexually active women are not using contraception even though they do not wish to become pregnant. Do we know whether and why current services are not meeting the population's needs? The published literature describes:

- inadequate services: access and availability limited, competition between different providers (e.g. GP surgeries and local family planning clinics)

- inadequate training of staff
- mismatch between services provided and the needs of subgroups of the population
- lack of knowledge of 'users' of services and non-users of available methods
- negative attitudes – of women and men to using contraception
- poor circumstances of many youngsters who have unplanned pregnancies, low self-esteem, adoption of risky lifestyle behaviour.

Setting criteria and standards

An audit project in North Staffordshire looked at the standards of contraceptive service care for young people. The standard set was that all teenagers who had a live birth or termination of pregnancy should receive contraceptive advice before leaving hospital, after the birth or termination.[9]

Comparing performance with standards

Ninety-four per cent of teenagers who had a live birth and 47% of those who had a termination of pregnancy received contraceptive advice before they were discharged from hospital. Several teenagers reported that they had not had enough time to ask questions.

Changes were made

Hospital staff introduced new procedures especially for teenagers having terminations of pregnancy who were treated as day cases. Changes were also triggered in primary care and family planning clinics to provide more consistent and more readily available contraceptive care and services.

Linking structure, process and outcome for an audit topic

If you are a practitioner with a special interest (PwSI), you will probably be expected to present the results of a substantial audit that spans the way you operate your special interest, each year. You will discuss the results with an expert in your special interest such as a hospital consultant, to demonstrate that you are competent to practise as a PwSI.

It will probably suit your purpose to organise an audit that combines aspects of the structure, process and outcomes of your special interest area. These might be:

- *structure*: premises or facilities
- *process*: communication (with colleagues or patients), record keeping
- *outcomes*: health gains or improvements in the way care is received by patients who have been under your care as a PwSI.

Judging how well you have performed an audit

Once you have completed an audit or a plan for an audit, use the criteria in Box 2.10 to check that you have been thorough and got the most out of the audit exercise.

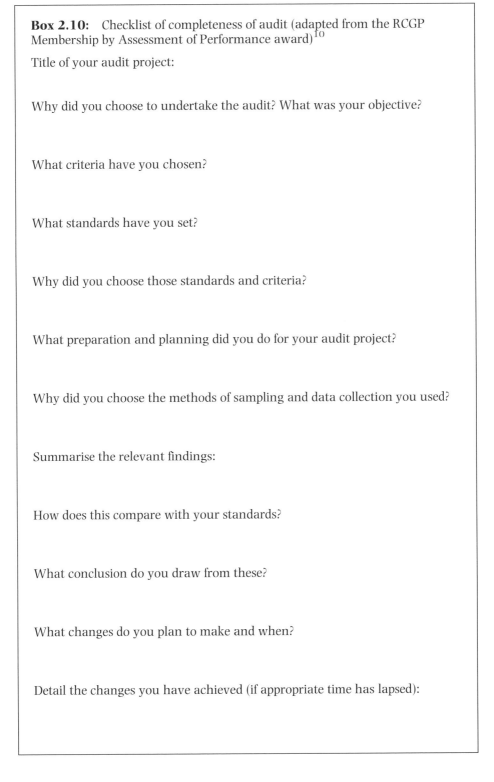

Box 2.10: Checklist of completeness of audit (adapted from the RCGP Membership by Assessment of Performance award)[10]

Title of your audit project:

Why did you choose to undertake the audit? What was your objective?

What criteria have you chosen?

What standards have you set?

Why did you choose those standards and criteria?

What preparation and planning did you do for your audit project?

Why did you choose the methods of sampling and data collection you used?

Summarise the relevant findings:

How does this compare with your standards?

What conclusion do you draw from these?

What changes do you plan to make and when?

Detail the changes you have achieved (if appropriate time has lapsed):

References

1   Chambers R, Drinkwater C and Boath E (2003) *Involving Patients and the Public. How to do it better* (2e). Radcliffe Medical Press, Oxford.

2   Blaxter L, Hughes C and Tight M (1996) *Research Methods in Primary Care*. Radcliffe Medical Press, Oxford.

3   General Practitioners Committee/The NHS Confederation (2003) *New GMS Contract. Investing in general practice*. British Medical Association, London.

4   www.gpaq.info

5   www.cfep.net

6   National Patient Safety Agency (NPSA) (2004) *Introduction to 7 Steps for Patient Safety*. NPSA, London. www.npsa.nhs.uk

7   Walsh K (2004) Appraisal and revalidation: how bmjlearning.com has helped. *Clinical Governance Bulletin*. **5(4)**: 5–6.

8   www.nhsleadershipqualities.nhs.uk/assessment.asp

9   Chambers R and Milsom G (1995) *Audit of Contraceptive Services in Mid and North Staffordshire in Secondary Care, Primary Care and the Community*. Keele University, Staffordshire.

10 Royal College of General Practitioners (2003) *Membership by Assessment of Performance*. Royal College of General Practitioners, London.

3

Quality, audit and evaluation

Impact of audit

It is often easier to audit structures (e.g. premises, records, workforce characteristics) and processes (e.g. practice procedures, medical interventions) than outcomes (e.g. impact of care or services). It may be many years before the impact or outcomes of care such as lengthening lifespan can be measured. There may be confounding factors that have contributed to bringing about the improvements. The outcome may be an absence of illness or harm which is impossible to identify accurately, e.g. prevention of pregnancy or a sexually transmitted infection; rather than a positive health gain.

Much will depend on how the objectives of the audit were phrased to ensure that the audit was targeted at a problem in the right way to result in action leading to effective change. Audit may be targeted at identifying where change is required for managerial purposes (e.g. feeding back information on prescribing or referrals to primary care organisations (PCOs) in relation to commissioning), to obtain better provision from, for example, community or secondary care, for practice services or procedures, or for individuals to change how they work. Each requires a different format and separate way of analysing and reporting the information.

In assessing the overall impact of a particular treatment or service, you should consider the four dimensions of effectiveness, value, impact and efficiency as well as the public's or particular patients' preferences and views.

- *Effectiveness* is the extent to which a treatment or other healthcare intervention achieves a desired effect.
- *Value* is a judgement made by an appropriate group as to how valuable that effect is in one patient relative to the value of other treatments. Quality adjusted life years (QALYs) are one way of measuring value.
- *Impact* is the value of an effect weighted for the degree of effectiveness. A treatment or intervention with a high impact will be highly effective, and the effect will be considered very valuable by most people (for example extend life by a reasonable amount, good reduction of pain etc).
- *Efficiency* is the cost of the treatment or intervention for a particular level of impact.

Assessing quality

Defining quality depends very much on whose perspective of quality you are using or who is describing the extent or nature of the impact. The aspects of care that are most highly valued by patients are:[1]

- availability and accessibility of care – appointments, reasonable waiting times, good physical access, ready telephone access

- technical competence – health professionals' knowledge and skills, effectiveness of professionals' treatment
- communication – time to listen and explain, give information and share in decisions
- interpersonal factors such as a health professional being humane, caring, supportive and trustworthy
- good organisation of care – continuity, co-ordination, location of services.

Using audit to assess quality

If you are considering the quality of care that a patient is receiving when they are being treated you should question whether the treatment is:

- available
- available to all patients on an impartial basis (whatever their gender, age, social class, ethnicity, religion, postcode of their residence)
- the right one
- acceptable to the patient (e.g. type of treatment, frequency, fits with their religious or ethical beliefs)
- delivered at the right time
- delivered in the right way
- achieving the desired effects or outcomes
- achieving the desired outcomes with minimum effort, expense and waste.[2]

You could audit any or all of these items if you wanted to focus on the quality of any treatment, for instance for leg ulcers, or asthma.

Quality of healthcare has been subdivided into eight components:

- equity
- access
- acceptability and responsiveness
- appropriateness
- communication
- continuity
- effectiveness
- efficiency.[3]

You might use some of these components organised in a matrix as in Box 3.1 as a way of ordering your approach to auditing a particular topic. Include, say, four aspects of quality on the vertical axis, with structure, process and outcome on the horizontal axis. In this example, you could generate up to 12 aspects of quality for undertaking an audit in a clinical field. You might then focus on several of these aspects to look at the quality of patient care or services from various angles.

For example, if you were carrying out an audit of the care you provide for people with diabetes, you might look at:

- whether patients from hard-to-reach groups such as young people have good access to your routine diabetic clinic (structure; access)
- the process of communicating results to patients (process; communication)
- the extent to which a GP and nurse stick to the diabetic protocol at successive consultations, providing consistent advice (process; continuity)

- whether the management of diabetes (as measured by patients' HbA_{1c} results) is equally as effective for patients attending routine GP surgeries or nurse-run chronic disease clinics (outcome; HbA_{1c} results).

For each of these components you would organise a separate but linked audit. You should be able to organise an audit protocol that scrutinises the computer records of consultations to gain information about the way results are communicated and HbA_{1c} levels at the same time. You will have to survey patients to investigate their views about access and communication. You should be able to organise the data collection so that you perform it once to cover more than one aspect of quality in this way.

Box 3.1: Matrix for quality assessment of care you provide for people with diabetes

	Structure	**Process**	**Outcome**
Access	Diabetes clinic		
Communication		Results	
Continuity		Clinic protocol	
Effective care			HbA_{1c}

Quality assurance

Quality assurance consists of quality measurement and quality improvement. Continuous quality improvement and total quality management are both umbrella terms that have become devalued over time by their multiple interpretations. Quality assurance has been defined as 'the measurement of actual quality of care against pre-established standards, followed by the implementation of corrective actions to achieve those standards'.[4]

Evaluating your audit effort

Evaluation is an essential component of any programme or service – incorporate it into any plan from the beginning. Time and effort spent on evaluation should be in proportion to the activity that is being evaluated. Keep it as simple as possible and avoid wasting resources on unnecessarily bureaucratic evaluation.[5]

Evaluation sets out measurable targets and timescales that are realistic for the particular context and problems of the population group you are auditing. Agree on short-, medium- and longer-term outcomes with all the 'stakeholders' before the audit begins.[6] There are always risks that other factors may crop up that are not under your control, and that the outcomes you originally expected if your project worked well are no longer viable or possible.

Evaluate the quality of the audit you are undertaking to ensure that the approach you take is appropriate and relevant to your patient population:

- agree what criteria you will use for the outcome of the audit, e.g. that it measured what it set out to measure
- invite external review either from an independent person or by comparing what you have done against external standards
- use peer review from neighbouring practices or comparison with their standards, or the results of other audits collected by the PCO
- assess how well you have done in one area. You might include one or more item: activity, personnel, provision of service, organisational structure or objectives in your evaluation.

Setting up evaluation of any changes you make is complicated by the fact that the outcome may be dependent on many factors other than your own initiative, or it may take a long time to see results.

What to evaluate

Evaluate your audit work to ensure that the investment of time and effort was worthwhile. You might assess whether:

- everyone participated in the actual audit measuring their performance
- the objectives of the audit were well phrased, simple, measurable, achievable, realistic and timely
- everyone supported and adhered to any changes made as a result of audit
- proposed changes were implemented
- staff or your training needs that were identified were addressed
- the need for any further audits was indicated, and if so whether they were undertaken
- the topic that was audited was important enough to have justified the effort and cost
- there was good leadership of the audit group and practice team
- the method used was appropriate for the purpose and objective(s) of the audit
- findings were conveyed to everyone that they affected, and results were discussed
- there was an emphasis on teamworking and support
- the practice culture and environment were conducive to conducting audit
- the quality of patient care improved
- acceptable outcomes were used to measure any interventions or changes to patient care.[7]

Design the evaluation so that you:

- specify exactly what part of the audit you are evaluating using the list above or additional areas
- set priorities against what you need to achieve and the time and resources available
- obtain agreement from the audit team on the nature and scope of the task
- describe the expected impact of the programme or activity and who will be affected
- define the criteria of success – these might relate to structure, process or outcome
- identify the information required to demonstrate what the team achieved in the audit. The information required might include: observing behaviour, data from existing records, prospective recording by the subjects of the programme or by the recipients and staff of the activity

- determine how long it will take overall and what you will do by what time
- decide who collects the information about the audit or the changes and the respective deadlines for collecting the data
- review and refine the objectives of the audit and check that they are appropriate for the outcomes and impact you expect.

Assessing significant event analysis

You could use the schedule in Box 3.2 to assess one of your significant event analyses. You could undertake this yourself or with practice colleagues, or invite an assessor from another practice or the PCO to look at your audit.[8]

Box 3.2: Significant event analysis assessment schedule[8]

Tick those that apply*

1 What happened:
- has personal impact ☐
- is important to the individual or organisation ☐
- causes reflection ☐

2 Why did it happen?
- a clear reason was sought ☐

3 Demonstrated insight?
- those involved became aware of previous suboptimal care ☐
- the decision-making process was altered ☐
- awareness of 'risk' was demonstrated ☐
- level of personal responsibility was linked to circumstances ☐

4 Was change implemented?
- yes – describes the implementation of relevant change ☐
- no – risk of similar significant event unlikely ☐
- no – unable to influence change but suggestions for change given ☐

* You could modify this from the original simple yes/no score to a Likert scale of: excellent, well done, satisfactory, poorly done, very poorly done.

Other models of evaluation

A variety of other evaluation models exist to help teams set their aims, measures and targets and then plan the introduction of changes that will result in improvement. RAID is another model for evaluation and change.[5] RAID stands for:

- **R**eview: look at the current situation and prepare the organisation for change
- **A**gree: ensure that staff are signed up to the proposed changes
- **I**mplement: put in place the proposed changes
- **D**emonstrate: show that the changes have made improvements.

Other approaches include needs assessments, economic evaluation, evaluation of how well an initiative has been implemented.[9]

References

1 Roland M (1999) Quality and efficiency: enemies or partners? *British Journal of General Practice.* **49**: 140–3.

2 Newcastle-under-Lyme Primary Care Trust (2004) *Clinical Audit Policy.* Newcastle-under-Lyme PCT, Staffordshire.

3 Maxwell R (1984) Quality assessment in health. *British Medical Journal.* **288**: 1470–2.

4 Vuori H (1989) Research needs in quality assurance. *Quality Assurance in Health Care.* **1(2/3)**: 147–59.

5 Wood L (2001) *Review, Agree, Implement, Demonstrate.* National Clinical Governance Support Team, Leicester.

6 Pawson R and Tilley N (2000) *Realistic Evaluation.* Sage, London.

7 Chambers R and Wakley G (2000) *Making Clinical Governance Work for You.* Radcliffe Medical Press, Oxford.

8 Bowie P, McKay J and Lough M (2003) Peer assessment of significant event analyses: being a trainer confers an advantage. *Education for Primary Care.* **14**: 338–44.

9 Lazenbatt A (2002) *The Evaluation Handbook for Health Professionals.* Routledge, London.

4

Promoting change after audit

It is highly likely that you will be able to identify some potential improvements after analysing an audit. But only make changes if they are warranted and agreed by those participating in an audit. If the improvement will not make much difference, concentrate your efforts elsewhere. Don't make changes just for the sake of it or to follow a fashion.

Change happens all the time. Think how you can help to make transitions occur more smoothly by:

- deciding on what needs to be changed, through gathering evidence
- sharing the responsibility for identifying the problem and finding the solutions, so that everyone feels part of the process (ownership)
- building in plenty of time to discuss the planned changes so that everyone feels that they have had a chance to put their point of view
- making the changes in small steps
- giving plenty of support in monitoring progress
- giving feedback so that everyone knows how the changes are progressing and what their part in them means to the whole
- celebrating completion and continuing monitoring to prevent backsliding!

Despite the excitement that changes can bring we tend to resist change. To improve quality, change is inevitable.

Think about four levels of change:

- do you need to do something new?
- should you do things differently – change a system or process?
- should you do something different – change the purpose?
- do you need to stop doing something – does the service or organisation need to exist at all?

Identifying how people react to change

Some people embrace change eagerly; others resist it steadfastly. Everyone passes through stages in accepting change (*see* Figure 4.1), some more quickly than others.

Factors that influence how change is perceived and how much resistance occurs include:

- whether change was imposed or agreed voluntarily
- whether the need for change was recognised
- how seriously the change affects the individual
- how the individuals responded to change previously
- how much support is available during and after the change.

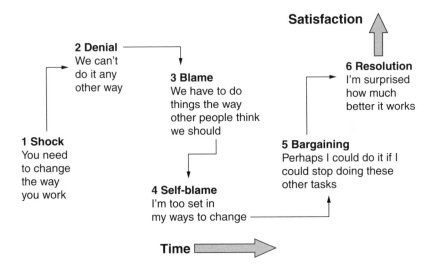

Figure 4.1:   Stages in the response to change

If the individuals involved are dissatisfied with the present situation as outlined by the audit, they will be more willing to make changes.

How to introduce change

Ensure that you map out a clear plan for change in behaviour or procedures so that everyone knows where he or she is heading and the steps they need to take. Break the change down into its constituent parts as in Figure 4.2.

You may find that some of the changes have already occurred as part of doing the audit. For example, a recently introduced protocol may have been poorly followed because people were still not remembering to use it. Auditing how well the protocol was followed reminds people to adhere to it. They use the protocol and become more familiar with the requirements, so that it becomes an automatic procedure rather than a new one. You may find that data-gathering leads to more precision in recording. Or the discussions before and after doing the audit lead to changes in behaviour as people realise the consequences of their actions or omissions more clearly.

To manage change successfully you can:

- ensure that people understand and accept why the change is necessary
- set realistic timescales
- communicate clearly what is to happen
- prevent or correct rumours that mislead people about the purpose or actions required
- consult the staff and other colleagues constantly
- estimate the resources needed
- plan to make small changes that show improvements at an early stage, so that people feel rewarded for their efforts
- make sure that people realise that they have a role (or job) after the change.

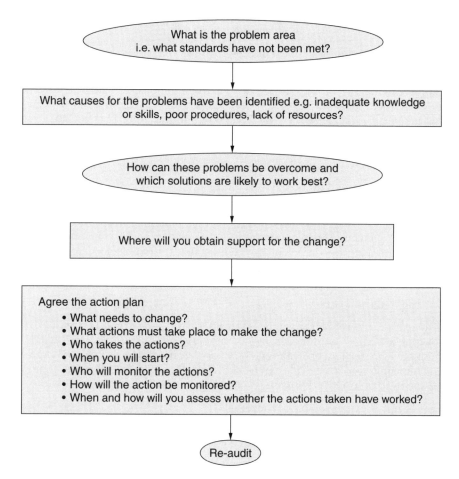

Figure 4.2: Making a change

Avoiding common pitfalls

If people think the job that they do will change into something they dislike, or that the job will disappear altogether, you will have great difficulty gaining their co-operation. Similarly, do not underestimate the amount of continuous information, support and encouragement that is needed for successful change, to prevent the action plan from being derailed or subverted. Simply circulating information about the proposed change is not enough.

Other mistakes that are common in relation to making change happen include:

1 failure to anticipate the knock-on effects of one change on another area

Example: you may ask a practice nurse to include some extra activities in her workload to meet the required standards of the criteria, but this takes her away from other essential duties. You must consider who will do the work she will no longer have time to do, whether there are other tasks that she can stop or delegate to make time for the new actions, or whether you need more nurse hours.

2   one change interfering with another in complex organisations

Example: spirometry testing is one of the requirements of the chronic disease management criteria for chronic obstructive pulmonary disease. The practice nurse is asked to go on a course to learn how to do this and upgrade her asthma management skills. Following the results of another audit, it is decided that she also needs training to manage reviews of people with chronic heart disease, and there is acrimonious disagreement between the two doctors leading each chronic disease area as to the priority that she gives to each activity.

3   the action is hijacked by vested interests

Example: the lead clinician for the hypertension and chronic heart disease domains has been offered automated blood pressure equipment that is linked into the computer system. A pharmaceutical company that wants him to do some post-marketing studies will supply the equipment. To accommodate the new devices, he now wants to change the blood pressure monitoring system that was agreed by all involved after a previous audit.

4   the diagnosis or solution is wrong

Example: an audit shows that few people attend the appointments sent out to them for review of their asthma. It is agreed that one of the practice nurses will phone patients who need an asthma review. However, the practice nurse only works in the mornings and few people can be contacted then. She feels that her time could be spent more usefully doing nursing tasks.

5   the change is overtaken by new events

Example: many practices have put into place careful procedures for monitoring warfarin anticoagulation treatment. If the new oral treatment being piloted that does not require monitoring is successfully introduced,[1] the actions following auditing of the standards of care for this programme will not be required.

6   a lack of ownership or commitment (especially if key people leave)

Example: an enthusiastic member of staff undertakes extra IT training through gaining a European Computer Driving Licence. She sets up excellent recording and reporting schemes in the practice, but is then lured away by higher status and more money now that she has the extra qualification. No-one else knows how to maintain the schemes and they fall into disuse.

7   the change cannot be implemented because of a lack of resources

Example: following an audit of the care of people with mental health problems you identify a need for advice on financial benefits and social care. You offer accommodation for a social worker or Citizens Advice Bureau worker in the practice premises, but no-one is available. The feedback from patients after referral to social services or to the Citizens Advice Bureau shows that long waiting lists for any advice deters them from seeking help. The team feels disinclined to identify the needs of patients and refer them, if there is no possibility of them receiving help in the near future.

Identifying resistance to change

It helps to be able to recognise types of resistance to change[2] and how you can tackle them (*see* Table 4.1).[2]

Table 4.1: Types of resistance to change

Types of resisters	What you can do
The *victim* is helpless in the face of events	Give the *victim* support and help in standing up for themselves, taking ownership of the change for his/herself
The *rebel* refuses to do things because someone in authority has suggested it	Enlist the *rebel* in helping to lead the changes
The *oppressor* persecutes the victims	Help the *victim* to stand up for his/herself and become self-motivating
The *rescuer* takes the side of the victim against the oppressor	Encourage both individual action and co-operation in teams. Break up colluding subversion by altering work patterns and changing working partners

For change to be successful, the perceived benefits must outweigh the perceived barriers. The individuals involved will take into account the attitudes of others to any changes and enthusiasts can carry others along with them. The individuals also have to believe that they are able to make the changes themselves before they accept that they will make the changes.

Recognise the signs of resistance to change in yourself and in others if you:

- use outdated methods
- avoid new duties or ways of working
- control and resist the change
- play the victim and use others to do the new work
- wait for someone else to implement it
- stop being able to do your present work properly.

Stress levels are often high in general practices, especially when multiple changes are occurring. This can increase resistance to change. Getting people to work together and support each other reduces their stress levels and levels of resentment. Look at Chapter 3 for ways to evaluate teamworking.

Building a learning culture

People become more inclined to change, learn and innovate if they perceive that their environment is one in which constant learning (and change) is occurring. Make sure that you:

- build innovation and flexibility into day-to-day functioning
- have regular reviews to extract learning from practical experience
- plan improvements for the future
- encourage innovation and creativity in *all* the staff

- encourage individuals' development
- review the practice or department's direction regularly as circumstances alter.

The evidence for successful methods of change is sparse. It is difficult to measure whether changes that occur are actually due to what you did, or occurred anyway, or were influenced by other external events. Look at the *Effective Health Care Bulletin* 'Getting Evidence into Practice' for ideas about what actually works.[3] They include among the strategies evaluated that:

- continuing medical education interventions were likely to be more successful if they included educational outreach, opinion leaders, patient-mediated interventions and reminders. Using more than one intervention method and using an assessment of the barriers to change increased success
- passive dissemination of guidelines was unlikely to work. Complex guidelines were less likely to be followed than simple ones. Guidelines could change clinical practice and were more likely to be effective if they took account of local circumstances, were disseminated by active educational activities and were reinforced by patient-specific reminders
- for health promotion activities, training had a small effect, while reminder systems, audit and feedback were generally effective
- mailed educational materials were generally ineffective at changing prescribing habits, but educational outreach and continuing feedback were successful
- computer-based reminder systems could lead to improvements in decisions about drug dosages, the provision of preventive care and the general clinical management of patients.

How to learn more about managing change

A useful resource appeared in *Bandolier*.[4] It contains a slide presentation that could be used as the basis for a workshop to examine the issues involved in implementing improvements in clinical practice. The summary concludes that:

1 implementing change is a complex, non-linear process. It is unlikely that the work will move forward in a logical sequence
2 time and resources are required to support the project activity
3 there is a need for flexibility because of the unexpected
4 good communications are essential to ensure that those affected by the work understand how the work is being handled and progressing.

References

1 Francis CW, Davidson BL, Berkowitz SD *et al.* (2002) Ximelagatran versus warfarin for the prevention of venous thromboembolism after total knee arthroplasty. *Annals of Internal Medicine.* **137(8)**: 648–55.

2 NHS National Institute for Clinical Excellence, Commission for Health Improvement, Royal College of Nursing and University of Leicester (2002) *Principles for Best Practice in Clinical Audit.* Radcliffe Medical Press, Oxford.

3 NHS Centre for Reviews and Dissemination (1999) Getting evidence into practice. *Effective Health Care Bulletin.* **5(1)**. Royal Society of Medicine Press, London.

4 www.jr2.ox.ac.uk/bandolier/booth/mgmt/Better3.html

Part 2

Worked examples of audits: templates for you

Worked examples of audits: templates for you

You will learn more about clinical audit by doing it than reading about it. We have included two worked examples of audits in general practice from 14 fields. They are mainly based on the clinical fields of the General Medical Services (GMS) contract for general medical practices,[1] but some concern non-clinical components of the practice organisation.

The introduction to each template indicates how the topic or field is important: whether it (1) is high risk, (2) is high volume, (3) causes concern or (4) is high cost.

The criteria and standards of ten of the clinical fields are extracted from the Quality and Outcomes Framework (QOF) of the GMS contract;[1] or if the clinical topic is not included in the QOF, from a reputable source. For each audit we suggest five steps in the design of an audit.

We remind you to decide who will analyse the data and feed back the results. The same person or others in the team will decide what changes are needed and negotiate how change is made. Then all that is left is the re-audit.

You can simply read through the 28 worked examples of audit and use the content of the templates to guide you in constructing your own audit. Or choose one or more topics included here and mirror the audit template in your own practice with your own team.

As you encourage clinical audit and reflection in your practice, the benefits to patient care will become increasingly obvious, and your reward points from the QOF should shoot up.

Good luck.

Reference

1 General Practitioners Committee/The NHS Confederation (2003) *New GMS Contract. Investing in general practice.* British Medical Association, London.

Audit template

Asthma 1: diagnosis

Select the topic and review the literature

An audit topic should concern an area that has at least one of the following characteristics:

(1) high risk
(2) high volume
(3) causes concern
(4) high cost

Inadequately treated patients run a higher risk of exacerbations (1). National prevalence is around 8% so that large numbers of patients (2) will be on the practice register for the Quality and Outcomes Framework (QOF). Patients, especially children and young adults, labelled incorrectly as having asthma, may suffer harm (3), e.g. by being refused access to certain employment opportunities.[1] Adequate treatment is expensive, but inadequate treatment is just as costly (4).

Criteria

The QOF states that the practice can show that:

Criteria	Maximum threshold (minimum 25%)	Points
Patients aged 8 years and over, diagnosed with asthma after 1 April 2003, have had the diagnosis confirmed with peak flow measurement or spirometry	70%	15

New peak flow meters issued in 2004 read accurately across the whole range of measurement and may give different readings from the traditional Wright peak flow meter. Patients who have personalised asthma plans will need their personal best peak flow and action levels recalculated when they are issued with a new peak flow meter. Aim to change all your patients over to the new peak flow meter gradually over the next 12 months when the peak flow meter needs replacing or at an asthma review.[2]

Standards

Standards should be:

- realistic
- measurable
- achievable
- agreed

You may want to start with lower targets than the maximum threshold of the QOF if you have only recently been able to enter lung function measurements into a coded computer template. When you repeat the audit, set your standards higher than the last time.

Designing the audit

Selection of sample

You might choose to look at all new entries onto the practice asthma register since 1 April 2003.

Prospective or retrospective

The audit has to be retrospective because of the nature of the data.

Collecting the data

- If you have not been recording lung function values into a Read-coded template, this has to be done now.
- Run a search every three to six months to establish how near you are to your target.
- List the patient identities of those with a diagnosis of asthma and no computer record of lung function.
- The health professional lead will have to search the free text entries on computer or the written medical notes for the lung function tests that are missing.

Who will collect the data?

- A member of the primary care team trained in audit searches.
- The health professional lead on asthma management.

Resources required to complete the audit

- Designated time to do the searches.
- The health professionals responsible for the diagnosis and reviews of patients with a diagnosis of asthma need training and enough time to enter the lung function tests into the template.
- The lead clinician needs designated time to search the computer free text or written medical records for lung function recordings. This will be intensive work the first time, but few results should be missing after lung function tests are entered routinely.
- Time is required for all the relevant members of the practice team to meet and discuss the findings and agree the way in which changes will be implemented.

Who will analyse and present the data?

The lead clinician on asthma management is ideal.

Feeding back and negotiating change

You should look at the changes required with all the practice team members involved. For example, the audit may indicate:

- a lack of training in the use of the computer, so that lung function tests are not recorded in a retrievable form. Training is arranged by the practice manager for all staff who are carrying out lung function tests
- problems with inadequately maintained or calibrated equipment, so that tests are not completed at the time of diagnosis. The primary care organisation is approached to purchase a calibration device for the spirometer. The cost is shared between practices carrying out spirometry and the device is loaned to practices to calibrate their equipment regularly
- it is difficult to persuade patients to attend for lung function tests when they are well, and not suitable to test them during exacerbations. Discussions are initiated with the primary care organisation and local pharmacies, to see if lung function tests could be carried out when patients collect their prescriptions for inhalers as an enhanced pharmacy service.

Influencing changes resulting from the audit

The lead clinician is responsible for monitoring whether the changes agreed are followed through. He or she may need to support training or education e.g. in correct management, coding or in patient information and the queries arising from that process.

Planning to re-audit

Have a timetable of planned audits, so that this regular audit does not clash with others. Revise the standards ready for the next round, taking into account the changes that have been agreed.

References

1 Chambers R, Wakley G and Pullan A (2004) *Demonstrating Your Competence 4: Respiratory Disease, Mental Health, Diabetes and Dermatology.* Radcliffe Publishing, Oxford.

2 http://devices.mhra.gov.uk/mda/mdawebsitev2.nsf/0/DE2B2304788A7AC280256EA8003D47CE?OPEN

Audit template

Asthma 2: reviews

Select the topic and review the literature

An audit topic should concern an area that has at least one of the following characteristics:

(1) high risk
(2) high volume
(3) causes concern
(4) high cost

Review patients with asthma (1 and 2) regularly. Where asthma is controlled well, consider stepping down treatment. The aim is to maintain the patient at the lowest dose of inhaled steroid that controls the asthma (3). Reductions should be considered every three months (4), decreasing the dose by approximately 25–50% each time.[1] Reviews by community pharmacists can be a useful alternative or supplement to reviews by practice nurses or GPs.[2]

Criteria

The QOF states that the practice can show that it has:

Criteria	Maximum threshold (minimum 25%)	Points
Patients on the asthma register who have had an asthma review in the last 15 months	70%	20

Consider using a template for recording the review to ensure that the same things are done each time. As well as smoking history and influenza immunisation records, this might include those items in Box 1.

Box AT1: Template items for asthma review

Symptoms

Difficulty sleeping because of asthma	Yes	No
Daytime symptoms of cough, wheeze, breathlessness, tight chest	Yes	No
Asthma interferes with normal activities	Yes	No

What treatment is actually in use?
Reliever: times/day

Steroid dose and times/day

Other medication:

Date of last asthma attack:

Did it require hospital treatment?   Yes   No

Date of last occasion oral steroid required:

Reduction of steroid therapy indicated?   Yes   No

Dose recommended and review date entered in repeat prescription list:

Standards

Standards should be:

*   realistic
*   measurable
*   achievable
*   agreed

Arrange a meeting between the pharmacists providing a review service and the practices involved, so that there are agreed standards and interchange of information. Start with much lower targets than the maximum QOF percentage if you have only just started to organise care in a systematic way.[3] When you repeat the audit, set your standards higher than the last time. The lower percentage set by the QOF takes account of the numbers of patients who do not attend for regular review.

Designing the audit
Selection of sample
If you just record whether patients on the asthma register have been reviewed, you would look at the total number. If you are checking to see if the review is done consistently well, look at sufficient numbers to convince your colleagues, e.g. 1 in 10.

Prospective or retrospective
The audit has to be retrospective because of the nature of the data.

Collecting the data

- You will be able to search for the data quickly and easily if reviews are always entered into a computer template. Everyone involved should know which code to enter.
- Run a search every three to six months to establish how near you are to your target percentage being reviewed.
- Select your predetermined sample and look at the template completion.

Who will collect the data?

- A member of the primary care team trained in audit searches.
- The lead professional for the asthma review programme.

Resources required to complete the audit

- Designated time to do the searches.
- The pharmacists, nurses or doctors responsible for reviews of patients with a diagnosis of asthma have had training and have enough time to enter the data into the template.
- The lead professional needs designated time to search the computer free text or written medical records for asthma review data. This should be a task of diminishing necessity.
- Time for all the relevant members of the asthma review team to meet and discuss the findings and agree the way in which changes will be implemented.

Who will analyse and present the data?

The lead professional for the asthma review team is ideal.

Feeding back and negotiating change

You should look at the changes required with all the team members involved. For example, the audit may indicate:

- not all the data for the reviews are recorded in a retrievable form. Some of the nurses responsible say that they do not have enough time, but on closer examination, it appears that this is due to poor training and lack of confidence in using the computer template. In one of the pharmacies, a computer failure meant that data was not entered. Arrange training in the use of the template and written back-up in the event of a computer failure
- a large number of patients fail to attend when invited for review. It is decided to add reviews by telephone in designated time for two nurses trained in asthma management[4]
- few patients had sufficient information recorded to establish if they were stable. No reductions in treatment were made. The lead professional for asthma reviews will

organise an education session for staff, patients and carers on asthma management.

Influencing changes resulting from the audit

The lead professional for asthma reviews is responsible for monitoring whether the changes agreed are followed through. He or she may need to support training or education, e.g. in correct management and coding.

Planning to re-audit

Re-audit in 4–6 months to establish if the changes are effective. If they are, annual audit will pick up any backsliding.

References

1 British Thoracic Society/Scottish Intercollegiate Guidelines Network (2004) *Revised British Guideline on the Management of Asthma.* www.brit-thoracic.org.uk/docs/asthmafull.pdf

2 www.psnc.org.uk/index.php?type=more_news&id=388

3 Chambers R, Wakley G and Pullan A (2004) *Demonstrating Your Competence 4: Respiratory Disease, Mental Health, Diabetes and Dermatology.* Radcliffe Publishing, Oxford.

4 Pinnock H, Bawden R, Proctor S *et al.* (2003) Accessibility, acceptability, and effectiveness in primary care of routine telephone review of asthma: pragmatic, randomised controlled trial. *British Medical Journal.* **326**: 477–9.

Audit template
Hypertension 1: identification

Select the topic and review the literature

An audit topic should concern an area that has at least one of the following characteristics:

(1) high risk
(2) high volume
(3) causes concern
(4) high cost

Hypertension is a major risk factor for stroke and heart attacks (1 and 3). Hypertension, currently defined as blood pressure above 140 mmHg (systolic) and/or 90 mmHg (diastolic), is a common problem (2).[1] In the Health Survey for England, for example, the prevalence of hypertension as reported in the *ABC of Hypertension*[1] was 3% in those aged under 40 years, 28% in those aged between 40 and 79 years, and 50% in those aged 80 years and older.[1] Patient numbers for hypertension will be large and the cost of treatment considerable (4).

Criteria

The QOF states that the practice can show that it has a:

Criteria	Maximum threshold (minimum 25%)	Points
Register of patients with established hypertension	In line with expected prevalence	9
Blood pressure recorded in the previous 9 months for patients on the register	90%	20

Standards

Standards should be:

* realistic
* measurable
* achievable
* agreed

Increasingly, blood pressure screening is carried out in a multiplicity of venues (from pharmacies to outreach services in leisure centres and supermarkets), to increase the identification of raised levels.[2,3] A single level needs repeating at least twice to demonstrate sustained hypertension and the need for treatment.[4,5] Look at the guidance for pharmacies, and arrange to meet local pharmacists who are offering the service and other local action groups providing outreach services to ensure a unified approach to information for patients.[2,3]

Designing the audit

Selection of sample

- Search for all the patients recorded as having hypertension.
- Indicators are based on practices running six-monthly reviews (try to organise every three months to allow for slippage). Aim to record all blood pressures at review as coded entries on the computer, so that they can easily be retrieved.

Prospective or retrospective

The audit has to be retrospective because of the nature of the data.

Collecting the data

- Run a search every three to six months to establish how near you are to your target.
- List the patient identities of those with a diagnosis and no computer record of blood pressure reading or a review.
- The health professional lead, or trained deputy, will have to search the free text entries on computer or the written medical notes, for the values that are missing.

Who will collect the data?

- A member of the primary care team trained in audit searches.
- The health professional lead on hypertension management.

Resources required to complete the audit

- Designated time to do the searches.
- The health professionals responsible for the diagnosis and reviews of patients with hypertension need to have training and have enough time to enter the coded entries on the computer.
- The lead clinician or deputy needs time to search the computer free text or written medical records for missing data (less time will be needed as more data are correctly entered).
- Time for all the relevant members of those involved in identifying hypertension to meet and discuss the findings and agree the way in which changes will be implemented.

Who will analyse and present the data?
The lead clinician on hypertension is ideal.

Feeding back and negotiating change
You should look at the changes required with all involved. For example, the audit may indicate:

- a lack of training in the use of the computer, so that blood pressure results are not recorded in a retrievable form. Computer training is required and extra computer equipment may be needed
- problems with inadequately maintained or calibrated equipment, so that readings are misleading. Discuss the equipment and calibration required with pharmacies and outreach services. Make a nominated person responsible for arranging the regular servicing of equipment[4]
- patients feel well so that they do not comply with treatment, or fail to attend for review. Plan patient education initiatives with all the partners in the campaign[2-4]
- blood pressure readings taken by agencies outside the practice, including patient self-recording, are poorly recorded, so that records are unrepresentative. Patients are encouraged to bring written readings with them to reviews so that the figures can be entered.

Influencing changes resulting from the audit
The lead clinician is responsible for monitoring whether the changes agreed are followed through.

Planning to re-audit
Have a timetable of planned audits, so that this regular audit does not clash with others. Revise the standards ready for the next round, taking into account the changes that have been agreed.

References
1 Beevers DG, Lip GYH and O'Brien E (2001) *ABC of Hypertension* (4e). BMJ Publishing Group, London.

2 Royal Pharmaceutical Society of Great Britain (2003) *Practice Guidance on Blood Pressure Monitoring.* www.rpsgb.org.uk/pdfs/bpmonitguid.pdf

3 www.bpassoc.org.uk

4 Wakley G, Chambers R and Ellis S (2004) *Demonstrating Your Competence 3: Cardiovascular and Neurological Conditions.* Radcliffe Publishing, Oxford.

5 Williams B, Poulter NR, Brown MJ *et al.* (2004) Guidelines for management of hypertension: report of the fourth working party of the British Hypertension Society, 2004–BHS IV. *Journal of Human Hypertension.* **18**: 139–85. www.hyp.ac.uk/bhs/pdfs/BHS_IV_Guidelines.pdf

Audit template
Hypertension 2: treatment

Select the topic and review the literature

An audit topic should concern an area that has at least one of the following characteristics:

(1) high risk
(2) high volume
(3) causes concern
(4) high cost

Reducing blood pressure (BP) from raised levels is an activity that benefits patients.[1] Controlled levels gain quality and outcome points in this domain, as well as in the diabetes, cardiovascular, transient ischaemic attack (TIA) and stroke domains, because of the importance of reducing risk (1 and 2).[2] Most patients receive only one antihypertensive drug, but studies show that most patients require combinations of antihypertensive medication to reduce their risk of adverse cardiovascular events (3).[3] Strokes, heart attacks and ischaemic damage are very costly both personally and to communities (4).

Criteria

The QOF states that the practice can show records for:

Criteria	Maximum threshold (minimum 25%)	Points
Hypertension: Last BP 150/90 mmHg or less measured in the previous 9 months	70%	56
TIA and stroke: Last BP 150/90 mmHg or less measured in the previous 15 months	70%	5
Coronary heart disease and left ventricular dysfunction: Last BP 150/90 mmHg or less measured in the previous 15 months	70%	19
Diabetes: Last BP 145/85 mmHg or less in previous 15 months	55%	17

Standards

Standards should be:

- realistic
- measurable
- achievable
- agreed

The standards above will be difficult to meet especially for those who have high levels before, and often after, treatment. You might think that these targets are much too high for your practice population and want to start with lower levels, e.g. the minimum threshold of 25%. When you repeat the audit, set your standards higher than the last time.

Ensure that your practice disease registers are as accurate as possible. Record as exemptions all those who refuse treatment, have contraindications or adverse reactions to treatment, and those poorly controlled on maximal treatment.

Designing the audit

Selection of sample

You might want to obtain maximal reward for your efforts by targeting those patients who appear on all the disease registers, or three out of four registers, omitting diabetes with its more stringent criteria.

Prospective or retrospective

The audit has to be retrospective because of the nature of the data.

Collecting the data

- If you have not been recording blood pressures into a Read-coded template, this has to be done as soon as possible. You will find trawling through paper records or free text for records of blood pressures too time consuming.
- Set your recalls for the hypertensive group at six monthly review, so that searches pick up the last reading in the previous nine months. Other domains can be set for an annual review.
- Run a search every three to six months to establish how near you are to your target.

Who will collect the data?

- A member of the primary care team trained in audit searches.

- A designated health professional should look at the clinical data for the patients who are above the criteria of a blood pressure of 150/90 mmHg.

Resources required to complete the audit

- Patient records kept contemporaneously on a computer system make this audit easy to complete, provided clinicians enter the data under the agreed Read codes.
- Designated time to do the searches.
- The health professional must have designated time to analyse the data and propose the necessary changes.
- Time for all the relevant members of the practice team to meet and discuss the findings and agree the way in which changes will be implemented.

Who will analyse and present the data?

The analysis involves a health professional looking at clinical or patient reasons for failure to achieve the required levels, and adding exception coding to patient records as necessary.

Feeding back and negotiating change

You should look at the changes required with all the practice team members involved. For example, the audit may indicate:

- a lack of appreciation by patients of the importance of treating hypertension. You may want to find, or write, an information leaflet, with reinforcement of the advice by the health professionals when medication is reviewed[1]
- deficiencies in recording blood pressures in the correct template. Remind everyone involved of the necessity for Read recording correctly (not in free text) and use computer prompts that pop up to remind people when they consult with patients
- poor techniques in measuring blood pressure, with variations between individuals.[1] This causes friction between prescribers and staff carrying out monitoring, each of whom blames the other for high readings. A non-judgemental and social occasion is arranged with good food where everyone watches a CD presentation of correct procedures, then practises on each other
- persistence of out-of-date and insufficient prescribing habits. The prescribing lead of the primary care organisation is asked to give a short presentation to several practices and then some scenarios are worked through in small groups to establish best practice.[3]

Influencing changes resulting from the audit

The lead clinician is responsible for monitoring whether the changes agreed are followed through. He or she may need to support training or education.

Planning to re-audit

Revise the standards ready for the next round, taking into account the changes that have been agreed.

References

1 Wakley G, Chambers R and Ellis S (2004) *Demonstrating Your Competence 3: Cardiovascular and Neurological Conditions*. Radcliffe Publishing, Oxford.

2 Williams B, Poulter NR, Brown MJ *et al.* (2004) Guidelines for management of hypertension: report of the fourth working party of the British Hypertension Society, 2004–BHS IV. *Journal of Human Hypertension*. **18**: 139–85. www.hyp.ac.uk/bhs/pdfs/BHS_ IV_Guidelines.pdf

3 Brown MJ, Cruickshank JK, AF Dominiczak AF *et al.* (2003) Better blood pressure control: how to combine drugs. *Journal of Human Hypertension*. **17**: 81–6. www.hyp.ac.uk/bhs/resources/ABCD.pdf

Audit template
Epilepsy 1: identifying patients

Select the topic and review the literature

An audit topic should concern an area that has at least one of the following characteristics:

(1) high risk
(2) high volume
(3) causes concern
(4) high cost

The QOF estimates that around five to ten people per thousand will be receiving treatment for epilepsy (2). Identifying and helping people with epilepsy to lead a full and productive lifestyle reduces costs in personal terms and to the nation (3 and 4).[1,2]

Criteria

The QOF states that the practice can produce a register for:

Criteria	Maximum threshold (minimum 25%)	Points
Patients aged 16 years and over, receiving treatment for epilepsy	Within expected prevalence	2

People who have had the diagnosis of epilepsy made but who are not on medication should not be included when producing the disease register for the contract.

Standards

Standards should be:

- realistic
- measurable
- achievable
- agreed

You want to include all those people with epilepsy who are on treatment, but exclude those not on treatment or receiving anti-epileptic drugs for other conditions.[1] You may want to talk to patient representatives or look at how Epilepsy Action suggests you approach people with epilepsy.[3,4] Health professionals should use a consulting style that enables the individual with epilepsy, and their family and/or carers as appropriate, to participate as partners in all decisions about their healthcare, and take into account their specific needs.[1] You do not want to suddenly make people feel that they *have* to stand up and be counted after trying to avoid identification or stigma, but that you want to be able to help them to manage their epilepsy in a way that benefits them most.

Designing the audit

Selection of sample

Include everyone delineated by the criteria.

Prospective or retrospective

The audit has to be retrospective because of the nature of the data.

Collecting the data

- Set up a system to capture data from secondary care, as some people will not be managed in primary care. A new diagnosis will usually be made by secondary care and the diagnosis needs to be highlighted and added to the disease register as the hospital letters arrive.
- Run a search to establish how near you are to your target with just the Read-coded diagnosis.
- Search for those on anti-epileptic medication and merge those on both lists.
- Make a separate list of those on anti-epileptic medication but no diagnosis of epilepsy (unless you are lucky enough to have a system that tells you the indication for all medication). The health professional lead will have to search the free text entries on computer, or the written medical notes, for the diagnosis.

Who will collect the data?

- A member of the primary care team trained in audit searches.
- The health professional lead on epilepsy.

Resources required to complete the audit

- Designated time for audit searches.
- Designated time for the health professional to search for the diagnosis of people on anti-epileptic medication.

- Training and time for a secretary or clerk to enter diagnoses and reviews of epilepsy from secondary care letters.

Who will analyse and present the data?

The lead clinician on epilepsy management is ideal.

Feeding back and negotiating change

Look at the changes required with all the practice team members involved. For example, the audit may indicate:

- poor recording of diagnosis of epilepsy (or possibly reluctance in the past because of stigma), so that the diagnosis has to be entered, after investigation, for many people who have no listed indication for their medication
- long delays between the discharge of people on anti-epileptic medication and the receipt by the practice of a letter from the hospital clinic. Representations are made to the clinic and the primary care organisation to try and improve the speed of communication. With practice, the clerical staff become adept at spotting the diagnosis on the hospital letters even when the doctors forget to highlight it
- evidence that some people with epilepsy resented the increased and unexpected interest from the practice. A patient information programme was started to advertise the advantages of better and individualised management plans, including advice on contraception, pregnancy, driving and employment.[1-3]

Influencing changes resulting from the audit

The lead clinician is responsible for monitoring whether the changes agreed are followed through.

Planning to re-audit

Re-audit in about three months to ensure that the changes have been made. Then a search should only need repeating at annual intervals to check that the prevalence rates in the practice are in accord with those of the QOF.

References

1 National Institute for Clinical Excellence (2004) *The Epilepsies: the diagnosis and management of the epilepsies in adults and children in primary and secondary care.* National Institute for Clinical Excellence, London. www.nice.org.uk/pdf/CG020NICEguideline.pdf

2 Wakley G, Chambers R and Ellis S (2004) *Demonstrating Your Competence 3: Cardiovascular and Neurological Conditions.* Radcliffe Publishing, Oxford.

3 Chambers R, Drinkwater C and Boath E (2003) *Involving Patients and the Public: how to do it better.* Radcliffe Medical Press, Oxford.

4 www.epilepsy.org.uk

Audit template

Epilepsy 2: management

Select the topic and review the literature

An audit topic should concern an area that has at least one of the following characteristics:

(1) high risk
(2) high volume
(3) causes concern
(4) high cost

Most practices are not providing structured care for people on treatment for epilepsy.[1] Contraception needs and advice about employment or driving are poorly covered. Those whose seizures are poorly controlled require referral for specialist assessment.[2] Patients with epilepsy should have a comprehensive care plan that is agreed between the individuals, their family and/or carers as appropriate, and primary and secondary care providers. The anti-epileptic drug (AED) treatment strategy should be individualised according to the seizure type, epilepsy syndrome, other medication and conditions, the individual's lifestyle, and preferences of the individual, their family and/or carers.[2]

Criteria

The QOF states that the practice can show the percentage of:

Criteria	Maximum threshold (minimum 25%)	Points
Patients on the epilepsy register with a seizure frequency recorded in the past 15 months	90%	4
Patients on the epilepsy register with a record of medication review in the past 15 months	90%	4
Patients on the epilepsy register who have been seizure free for the past 12 months, recorded in the past 15 months	70%	6

Exception reporting will be more common than with some other conditions. For example, it may be difficult to control seizures in people with brain damage, and some patients cannot tolerate the dose of medication that would be required to control their seizures.

Standards

Standards should be:

- realistic
- measurable
- achievable
- agreed

Ensure that the nurses and/or doctors who will be responsible have sufficient training and education about the management of epilepsy to maintain consistent standards of care. You might include in the annual review:[1]

- seizure type and frequency, including the date of the last seizure
- medication and dosage
- an agreed management plan for the next 12 months
- other issues such as:
  - contraception
  - pregnancy planning
  - employment
  - driving
- referral for specialist care if seizures are not controlled or for other advice.[2]

Most computer systems include a template for recording an epilepsy review. Decide who is responsible for recall and review, and discuss with patients whether they might prefer a telephone review if they have no current problems. Your standard will probably be low (perhaps 25%) initially, unless you have someone with a special interest in epilepsy in your practice.

Designing the audit

Selection of sample

Include everyone on the epilepsy register.

Prospective or retrospective

The audit has to be retrospective because of the nature of the data.

Collecting the data

- Set up a system to capture data from secondary care, as some people will not be managed in primary care. Confirmation of diagnosis will also be made in secondary care. Changes in medication, reviews and seizure frequency need to be highlighted and added to the template by a designated person as the hospital letters arrive.

- Run a search to establish how near you are to your target.
- Make a separate list of those who have had a medication review but have missing data in the epilepsy template. The health professionals responsible, or trained deputies, will have to search the free text entries on computer or the written medical notes for the information.

Who will collect the data?

- A member of the primary care team trained in audit searches.
- The health professionals involved in the management of epilepsy care.

Resources required to complete the audit

- Designated time for audit searches.
- Designated time for the health professionals to search for missing data.
- Time for the health professionals or trained deputies to enter data from the reviews of epilepsy from secondary care letters.

Who will analyse and present the data?

The lead clinician on epilepsy management is ideal.

Feeding back and negotiating change

Look at the changes required with all the practice team members involved. For example, the audit may indicate:

- resistance by patients who have well-controlled epilepsy, to the idea of medical reviews. Telephone reviews seemed a good idea, but few patients appear to be at home during the working hours of the nurse responsible. It is agreed to send a printed out template form to the patients who need review, with a covering letter asking them to complete it. They are asked to either return it to the surgery in the envelope supplied (for confidentiality) with their next prescription request, or to bring it to their review appointment
- difficulty in using the template for epilepsy reviews during consultations. The practice manager arranges further training for the health professionals
- lack of information in the letters from hospital clinics. Representations are made to the clinics and the primary care organisation to try to improve the quality of information
- long delays after referral for seizure control or advice (except for pre-pregnancy advice). This has meant that some patients are having a second review before the specialist has seen them, annoying the patients and wasting time. Representations are made to the primary care organisation to try to increase secondary care provision.

Influencing changes resulting from the audit

The lead clinician is responsible for monitoring whether the changes agreed are followed through.

Planning to re-audit

Re-audit in about six months to ensure that the changes have been made successfully. If so, repeat the search at annual intervals.

References

1   Wakley G, Chambers R and Ellis S (2004) *Demonstrating Your Competence 3: Cardiovascular and Neurological Conditions*. Radcliffe Publishing, Oxford.

2   National Institute for Clinical Excellence (NICE) (2004) *The Epilepsies. The diagnosis and management of the epilepsies in primary and secondary care*. NICE, London. www.nice.org.uk/pdf/CGO20NICEguideline.pdf

Audit template

Chronic obstructive pulmonary disease 1: smoking

Select the topic and review the literature

An audit topic should concern an area that has at least one of the following characteristics:

(1) high risk
(2) high volume
(3) causes concern
(4) high cost

Large numbers of diseases are smoking related (1 and 3) and cause an enormous cost to individuals, families and governments (4). Around a quarter of adults in the UK smoke more than 15 cigarettes a day (2). Helping people to stop smoking has many health benefits and reduces costs.[1,2] It gains quality and outcome points in chronic obstructive pulmonary disease (COPD), as well as in the domains listed below.

Criteria

The QOF states that the practice can demonstrate smoking status and smoking cessation advice in the following conditions:

Criteria	Maximum threshold (minimum 25%)	Points
COPD: smoking status recorded in previous 15 months	90%	6
COPD: smoking cessation advice recorded in the previous 15 months	90%	6
Asthma: smoking status recorded in previous 15 months (patients aged 14–19 years)	70%	6
Asthma: smoking status recorded in previous 15 months (patients aged 20 years and over)	70%	6
Asthma: smoking cessation advice recorded in the previous 15 months	70%	6
TIA and stroke: smoking status recorded in previous 15 months	90%	3

TIA and stroke: smoking cessation advice recorded in the previous 15 months	90%	2
CHD and LVD: smoking status recorded in previous 15 months	90%	7
CHD and LVD: smoking cessation advice recorded in the previous 15 months	90%	4
Hypertension: smoking status recorded in previous 15 months	90%	10
Hypertension: smoking cessation advice recorded in the previous 15 months	90%	10
Diabetes: smoking status recorded in previous 15 months	90%	3
Diabetes: smoking cessation advice recorded in the previous 15 months	90%	5

COPD = chronic obstructive pulmonary disease; TIA = transient ischaemic attack; CHD = coronary heart disease; LVD = left ventricular dysfunction.

Standards

> Standards should be:
> - realistic
> - measurable
> - achievable
> - agreed

The target standards above will be difficult to meet unless computerised recording has been occurring for some time. You might want to start at the basic level of 25% and gradually increase your standards as you repeat the audit.

Designing the audit

Selection of sample

You could obtain maximal reward for your efforts by targeting those patients who appear on all six registers, or tackle just the respiratory registers initially.

Prospective or retrospective

The audit has to be retrospective because of the nature of the data.

Collecting the data

- If you have not been recording smoking and advice on smoking cessation into a Read-coded template, this has to be done as soon as possible. You will find trawling through paper records for information too time consuming.
- Run a search every three to six months to establish how near you are to your target.

Who will collect the data?

A member of the primary care team trained in audit searches.

Resources required to complete the audit

- Patient records kept contemporaneously on a computer system, provided health professionals enter the data under the agreed Read codes when they consult.
- Designated time for the audit searches.
- Time for all the relevant members of the practice team to meet and discuss the findings and agree the way in which changes will be implemented.

Who will analyse and present the data?

Choose someone involved in the audit, or ask for a volunteer.

Feeding back and negotiating change

Look at the changes required with all the practice team members involved. The audit may indicate:

- a lack of retrievable recorded data in the computerised medical record. Ways to increase this include:
    - patients complete information sheets from which the data are entered into the computerised record by reception and clerical staff
    - at routine review of medication in any of these domains complete a computer template that includes smoking history and smoking cessation advice boxes
    - *all* members of the practice team learn how to enter the information about smoking quickly and correctly
- poor referral for smoking cessation advice. Boxes of leaflets or cards are usually available from smoking cessation services. If not, prepare your own information. Placed on every health professionals' desk and on the reception desk, they act as a reminder so that patients can be given information when required.

Influencing changes resulting from the audit

Make a member of the practice team, e.g. a practice nurse or an audit clerk, responsible for overseeing the necessary changes and promoting improvements.

Planning to re-audit

A timetable of planned audits prevents clashes with other audits. Revise the standards ready for the next round, taking into account the changes that have been agreed.

References

1   www.ash.org.uk/html/factsheets/html/fact11.html

2   Raw M, McNeill A and West R (1998) Smoking cessation guidelines for health professionals: a guide to effective smoking cessation interventions for the healthcare system. *Thorax.* **53 (suppl. 5, Part 1)**: 1–19.

Audit template
Chronic obstructive pulmonary disease 2: nebuliser treatment

Select the topic and review the literature

An audit topic should concern an area that has at least one of the following characteristics:

(1) high risk
(2) high volume
(3) causes concern
(4) high cost

Chronic obstructive pulmonary disease (COPD) is a major cause of death and disability (1).[1] In your primary care organisation there are likely to be 54–55 deaths from COPD each year compared with only 2–3 deaths per year from asthma (2 and 3). This common condition is under-diagnosed and the symptoms frequently minimised by people who fear that they will simply be given a lecture on their smoking habits.[2] Nebulised drugs are considerably more expensive than other forms of inhaled therapy.[3] Using nebuliser treatment wisely in COPD will reduce costs (4).

Criteria

You should only start long-term nebulised treatment in COPD after a full assessment. Many patients may achieve similar benefit by using a large volume spacer with high dose bronchodilator (up to eight puffs four times daily).[4]

Criteria for nebulised bronchodilator therapy	Possible standard
The patient has had a trial of drug administration via a large volume spacer[4]	90%
The patient has had a full assessment by a respiratory specialist or general practitioner (GP) with specific training[4]	90%

You would discourage patients from buying their own nebuliser without a proper assessment for long-term treatment – but some patients will do so anyway.

Standards

Standards should be:

- realistic
- measurable
- achievable
- agreed

You would usually be asked about nebulised treatment when patients are severely or very severely affected by their symptoms.[2] You cannot insist that all patients are assessed before they purchase a nebuliser, but good information for patients will help to prevent inappropriate purchases and prescriptions for nebulised drugs.

Designing the audit

Selection of sample

A practice will have small numbers of people starting nebulised bronchodilator treatment and could include every patient in, say, a 24-month period.

Prospective or retrospective

If the audit is retrospective, you may have difficulty establishing the facts. Find out if your criteria are contained in the reports from the local respiratory clinic. If they are not, you may have to discuss the wording of the reports with the consultant. If the information will be included in the future, plan your audit prospectively.

Collecting the data

- Each time a new request for nebulised bronchodilator medication is made, all prescribers record the patient's details.
- The patient's details are passed to the respiratory lead, who searches the record for the criteria.
- If the patient is not requesting a repeat of medication started in secondary care, the request for the medication is discussed with the patient before initiation.
- If no record of the criteria is found, and the patient is under the care of the specialist respiratory team, the respiratory lead writes to the clinic or hospital to establish if the criteria have been carried out but the information not sent to the GP.

Who will collect the data?

A designated health professional looks at the clinical data for the patients who have requested a new prescription for nebulised bronchodilators.

Resources required to complete the audit

- All prescribers must remember to record the patient identifier for any new prescription for nebulised bronchodilators.
- Designated time for the health professional to search the records, communicate with the secondary care respiratory team, analyse the data and propose the necessary changes.
- Time for all the relevant members of the practice team to meet and discuss the findings and agree the way in which changes will be implemented.
- Good relationships with the secondary care respiratory team.

Who will analyse and present the data?

Normally a health professional will lead on respiratory conditions. The data involved will require clinical knowledge initially.

Feeding back and negotiating change

You should look at the changes required with all the practice team members involved. The audit may indicate a lack of:

- appreciation by the secondary care respiratory team of the need to inform the responsible prescriber of the rationale for medication. Negotiate changes to the supply of information
- understanding of the relative benefits of spacers and nebulisers by patients, relatives or their healthcare attendants. Improve the information interchange about treatment.

Influencing changes resulting from the audit

The lead clinician is responsible for monitoring whether the changes agreed are followed through. He or she may need to feed back the results of the audit to the primary care organisation, including the prescribing lead, to help to improve communication between primary and secondary care.

Planning to re-audit

Plan to repeat the audit after the necessary changes are in place.

References

1   Calverley PMA and Walker P (2003) Chronic obstructive pulmonary disease. *The Lancet.* **362**: 1053–61.

2   Chambers R, Wakley G and Pullan A (2004) *Demonstrating Your Competence 4: Respiratory Disease, Mental Health, Diabetes and Dermatology.* Radcliffe Publishing, Oxford.

3 Joint Formulary Committee (2004) *British National Formulary. BNF 48*. British Medical
   Association and the Royal Pharmaceutical Society of Great Britain, London.

4 The British Thoracic Society (1997) COPD Guidelines Summary. *Thorax*. **52 (suppl. 5)**: S1–
   S32. www.brit-thoracic.org.uk/copd

Audit template

Coronary heart disease 1: confirmation of diagnosis of angina

Select the topic and review the literature

An audit topic should concern an area that has at least one of the following characteristics:

(1) high risk
(2) high volume
(3) causes concern
(4) high cost

National prevalence of coronary heart disease (CHD) is around 3–4%. According to the National Service Framework for CHD, there are 1.4 million people in the UK with angina and 300 000 patients a year experience a myocardial infarction (1 and 2). The costs in terms of lost working life, long-term disability and medical treatment are enormous (4).[1,2]

Angina may be suspected from clinical symptoms and relief by taking nitrates, but chest pain may be misdiagnosed causing long-term unnecessary disability (3 and 4).[3]

Criteria

The QOF states that the practice can show the percentage of:

Criteria	Maximum threshold (minimum 25%)	Points
Patients with a new diagnosis of angina after 1 April 2003 referred for exercise testing or specialist opinion	90%	7

From April 2003, all patients that you suspect on clinical grounds may have angina should now have that diagnosis confirmed before the diagnosis of angina is coded. If you keep computerised records, code only the *symptom* before confirmation, for example, as 'chest pain' and add your query 'angina' in free text. The QOF points are for the referral, but for best practice, also monitor when your referrals are seen.

Standards

Standards should be:

- realistic
- measurable
- achievable
- agreed

You want to aim at confirming all suspected angina, but recognise that some patients may be too frail for assessment. Exercise testing is not relevant in someone who has severe chronic obstructive pulmonary disease or severe osteoarthritis, but confirmation may still be required. Refer in three ways:

- to a 'rapid access chest pain clinic' (if available). This provides a quick answer and prevents unnecessary disability from fear when angina is not confirmed. Standards for the time between referral and being seen for assessment should be agreed between primary and secondary care
- you may initiate treatment in patients in whom the diagnosis is fairly certain, e.g. previous history of myocardial infarction, while awaiting assessment for treatment of worsening cardiac function in secondary care
- patients with a possible acute coronary syndrome (e.g. angina at rest, prolonged pain, recent severe worsening and frequency of chest pain) are referred as emergencies to secondary care.

Designing the audit

Selection of sample

Look at how to identify all patients with suspected angina. Referrals may be made through a secretary, or doctors may make referral direct through a website for the rapid access clinic.

Prospective or retrospective

The audit is both prospective – looking at what happens to those with suspected angina, and retrospective to ensure that confirmation of diagnosis since 1 April 2003 has been done.

Collecting the data

- Whoever makes the referral must be responsible for entering the patient identifier on a list held manually or on a computer. You might keep a record as in the table opposite.

Table AT1: Collection of data for referral of chest pain suspected as angina

Patient identifier	Date seen with chest pain	Date referred for diagnosis	Date diagnosis made	Diagnosis confirmed	Diagnosis code entered
				Yes/No	Yes/No

- Patients may attend secondary care direct with chest pain. Designate an individual with suitable training to collect the information about a suspected or confirmed diagnosis from hospital discharge forms.
- Conduct a search to identify all patients with a diagnosis of angina since 1 April 2003, and establish whether the diagnosis has been confirmed by exercise testing or consultant assessment.

Who will collect the data?

- Whoever makes the referral of suspected angina.
- The designated person collecting the data from hospital discharge forms.
- The designated person conducting audit searches.
- The designated health professional examining the past records of angina diagnoses for confirmation.

Resources required to complete the audit

- Designated time for the searches, collection of data, examination of past records from 1 April 2003.
- Time for discussion of the results and plans for any necessary changes.

Who will analyse and present the data?

The lead clinician on CHD management is ideal.

Feeding back and negotiating change

You should look at the changes required with all the practice team members involved. For example, the audit may indicate:

- delays in referral for chest pain because not all clinicians were aware of the procedure for rapid referral. The protocol is placed in the referral information pack for any doctors working in the practice (including GP registrars, locums, etc), and the secretary undertakes to remind doctors when necessary

- some patients were coded as having angina before confirmation. A few patients had had a diagnosis of angina on a hospital discharge letter without any supporting data; others had been entered by clinicians when they were sure on clinical grounds. Discussion with all the people involved in entering codes revealed that several did not understand the importance of avoiding this coding until the diagnosis was confirmed. They agreed to be more precise
- it was not always easy to find information about exercise testing in the patient record. It was agreed that this information would be entered as a code to help with searches.

Influencing changes resulting from the audit

The lead clinician is responsible for monitoring whether the changes agreed are followed through.

Planning to re-audit

This audit should be easier to repeat as the data will be mainly prospective and fewer in number. Re-audit the patients with a new coding for angina after six months, to establish that the changes agreed are being implemented.

References

1 Chambers R, Wakley G and Ellis S (2004) *Demonstrating Your Competence 3: Cardiovascular and Neurological Conditions*. Radcliffe Publishing, Oxford.

2 NHS Executive (2000) *National Service Framework for Coronary Heart Disease*. Department of Health, London.

3 Hopcroft K and Forte V (2003) *Symptom Sorter*. Radcliffe Medical Press, Oxford.

Audit template

Coronary heart disease 2: secondary prevention

Select the topic and review the literature

An audit topic should concern an area that has at least one of the following characteristics:

(1) high risk
(2) high volume
(3) causes concern
(4) high cost

Cardiovascular disease is a major cause of premature death in most European and North American populations (2). Secondary prevention of cardiovascular disease is started after an episode such as a myocardial infarction or angina, as individuals have demonstrated that they are at high risk (1). As well as recommending lifestyle changes and exercise rehabilitation, explain and prescribe preventive medication.[1,2] These drugs amount to a large proportion of the drug costs in primary care (4).

Criteria

The QOF states that the practice can show the percentage of:

Criteria	Maximum threshold (minimum 25%)	Points
Patients on a beta blocker	50%	7
Patients on an angiotensin converting enzyme (ACE) inhibitor	70%	7
Aspirin, alternative antiplatelet or warfarin recorded in the last 15 months	90%	7

From April 2003, all patients should either be recorded as being on these preventive drugs or recorded as having contraindications, adverse effects or refusal.

Standards

Standards should be:

- realistic
- measurable
- achievable
- agreed

The thresholds above recognise that many patients will have contraindications, such as asthma, to beta-blockers. Similarly, poor renal function may preclude use of ACE inhibitors.[1] You should record exceptions because of contraindications, intolerance or refusal.

   Low dose aspirin (75 mg per day) reduces the risk of another episode of myocardial infarction, stroke or other vascular thrombosis. The benefits outweigh the risks of both cerebral and gastrointestinal haemorrhage. Other antiplatelet drugs, e.g. clopidogrel, are very much more expensive, and are usually only used if aspirin is contraindicated. Indigestion is the commonest side-effect and, in patients at high risk of bleeding, aspirin can be combined with a proton pump inhibitor or misoprostol.[2] You could also check to ensure that aspirin is being used as first choice antiplatelet agent.

Designing the audit
Selection of sample
To maximise results for the effort, you may want to combine this group of patients with those on the register for stroke and transient ischaemic attacks, as many patients will appear on both registers.

Prospective or retrospective
The audit looks at retrospective data. The QOF looks at data since 1 April 2003.

Collecting the data
- Search for patients on the relevant disease registers, the relevant data on current medication and exclusion criteria.
- Make a list of patients on the register who do not have the relevant data entries, and examine the records for evidence of the data that have not been recorded in a retrievable form.

Who will collect the data?
- An audit clerk trained in searches.
- Staff trained in examining clinical entries, or clinicians.

Resources required to complete the audit

- Designated time for the searches, collection of data, and examination of past records from 1 April 2003.
- Time for discussion of the results and plans for any necessary changes.

Who will analyse and present the data?

The lead clinician on cardiovascular disease management is ideal.

Feeding back and negotiating change

You should look at the changes required with all the practice team members involved. For example, the audit may indicate:

- poor recording of exclusion criteria in a retrievable form. Many of the entries about adverse effects or contraindications have been recorded in free text or only in the paper record after house calls. It is agreed to record information about house calls on the computer. The computer program has recently had an upgrade with a pop-up screen for recording exclusions and automatically coding them, so this problem will be less likely to recur
- the searches have not differentiated between medication records of 'ever prescribed' and 'currently receiving'. The search criteria are modified. The audit clerk receives further training and better instruction in what the searches are intended to demonstrate
- many patients are not taking the medication regularly and are not current users at the time searches are performed. It is agreed that the practice nurses will use information leaflets to supplement and reinforce the advice they give at review appointments, and that doctors reviewing patients at home will supply a patient information leaflet.[3]

Influencing changes resulting from the audit

The lead clinician is responsible for monitoring whether the changes agreed are followed through.

Planning to re-audit

Re-audit in 4–6 months to ensure that the changes agreed have been carried out.

References

1 Chambers R, Wakley G and Ellis S (2004) *Demonstrating Your Competence 3: Cardiovascular and Neurological Conditions*. Radcliffe Publishing, Oxford.

2 Godlee F (ed.) (2004) *Clinical Evidence Concise* Issue 11. BMJ Publishing Group, London. www.clinicalevidence.com

3 www.prodigy.nhs.uk/PILs/

Audit template

Diabetes 1: reviews

Select the topic and review the literature

An audit topic should concern an area that has at least one of the following characteristics:

(1) high risk
(2) high volume
(3) causes concern
(4) high cost

Between 2 and 3% of people of all ages in the UK have types 1 or 2 diabetes (2). About 200 000 people are thought to have type 1 and more than a million have type 2 diabetes.[1] It is a chronic progressive disease that can result in premature death, ill-health and disability (1). The aim of medical management of diabetes is to prevent or delay the long-term complications of diabetes.[1] Biochemical screening can help to monitor the success of management and help to contain the high cost to individuals and society (4).[2-4]

Criteria

The QOF states that the practice can show the percentage of:

Criteria	Maximum threshold (minimum 25%)	Points
Patients on the diabetic register with a record of HbA_{1c} in the past 15 months	90%	3
Patients on the diabetic register with a last HbA_{1c} of 10 or less in the past 15 months	85%	11
Patients on the diabetic register with a last HbA_{1c} of 7.4 or less in the past 15 months	50%	16
Patients on the diabetic register with a record of serum creatinine in the past 15 months	90%	3
Patients on the diabetic register with cholesterol recorded in the last 15 months	90%	3
Patients on the diabetic register with last cholesterol 5 mmol/l or less in the previous 15 months	60%	6

Standards

Standards should be:

- realistic
- measurable
- achievable
- agreed

The lower thresholds for more stringent target levels of HbA_{1c} and cholesterol in the table above represent the difficulties of achieving such tight control.[2]

Designing the audit

Selection of sample

You might choose to look at all patients on the diabetic register since 1 April 2003, or choose a sampling method to identify a sufficient proportion of patients to convince your colleagues about your findings.

Prospective or retrospective

The audit has to be retrospective because of the nature of the data.

Collecting the data

- Run a search for the blood results in the above categories within the last 15 months for the patients on the diabetic register.
- List the patient identities of those on the register with no computer record of results.
- The health professional lead will have to search the free text entries on computer or written medical records for the tests or reviews that are missing.

Who will collect the data?

- A member of the primary care team trained in audit searches.
- The health professional lead on diabetes management.

Resources required to complete the audit

- Designated time for the searches.

- The health professionals responsible for the reviews of patients with diabetes or the recording of laboratory investigations must have had training and have enough time to enter the blood tests into the template.
- The lead clinician needs time to search the computer free text or written medical records for missing data.
- Time for all the relevant members of the practice team to meet and discuss the findings and agree the way in which changes will be implemented.

Who will analyse and present the data?

The lead clinician on diabetes management is ideal.

Feeding back and negotiating change

You should look at the changes required with all the practice team members involved. For example, the audit may indicate:

- many people on the diabetic register do not attend for their review appointments. An educational initiative is planned with two sessions for patients and carers to meet the specialist nurse in diabetes and hear about the management of diabetes. All members of the practice team encourage and remind patients about the importance of reviews. Information about the importance of monitoring is obtained and supplied to any patient with diabetes who attends for any reason
- difficulty in obtaining the data for people attending secondary care for monitoring. After representations to the hospital diabetic clinic and laboratory, the biochemical data are copied to the practice where it is entered by a trained data clerk
- during the discussion, anecdotal evidence is given that high readings do not always prompt changes in treatment. A separate audit is set up to monitor what changes are made at review appointments.

Influencing changes resulting from the audit

The lead clinician is responsible for monitoring whether the changes agreed are followed through. He or she may need to support training or education, e.g. in correct management, coding or in patient information and the queries arising from that process.

Planning to re-audit

Have a timetable of planned audits, so that this regular audit does not clash with others.

References

1 Chambers R, Wakley G and Pullan A (2004) *Demonstrating Your Competence 4: Respiratory Disease, Mental Health, Diabetes and Dermatology.* Radcliffe Publishing, Oxford.

2 Royal College of General Practitioners Effective Clinical Practice Programme (2002) *Clinical Guidelines for Type 2 Diabetes: management of blood glucose*. Royal College of General Practitioners, Effective Clinical Practice Unit, University of Sheffield. www.nice.org.uk/pdf/NICE_full_blood_glucose.pdf

3 British Medical Association, Board of Science and Education (2004) *Diabetes Mellitus: an update for healthcare professionals*. BMA Publications Unit, London. www.bma.org.uk

4 Scottish Intercollegiate Guidelines Network (2001) *Management of Diabetes – a national clinical guideline*. Royal College of Physicians of Edinburgh. **55**: 24–8. www.sign.ac.uk

Audit template

Diabetes 2: retinal screening and treatment

Select the topic and review the literature

> An audit topic should concern an area that has at least one of the following characteristics:
>
> (1) high risk
> (2) high volume
> (3) causes concern
> (4) high cost

For every 100 patients with diabetes with treatable eye disease, 55 individuals could be expected to become blind or severely visually impaired within 10 years if none of them were treated (1 and 3). If these 55 were detected and treated, only 13 individuals would be affected.[1] Studies have shown that screening for retinopathy in people with diabetes is cost-effective, as costs of screening and treatment are less than for dealing with blindness (4). Modern digital imaging has been shown to be reliable and effective.[2]

Criteria

The QOF states that the practice can show the percentage of:

Criteria	Maximum threshold (minimum 25%)	Points
Patients on the diabetic register with a record of retinal screening in the past 15 months	90%	5

In addition, you should ensure that the results of the screening have been acted upon and the necessary referrals organised.

Standards

Standards should be:

- realistic
- measurable
- achievable
- agreed

Prevention of blindness or loss of vision in people with diabetes requires:

- visual acuity in the corrected state, using a standard 6 m (or 3 m) Snellen chart. Use a pin hole if visual acuity is less than 6/9
- retinal examination by:
  - direct ophthalmology through pupils dilated with tropicamide
  - a combination of direct ophthalmology and slit lamp biomicroscopy
  - retinal photography through a non-mydriatic fundus camera.[1]

You may prefer to organise the retinopathy as an external service, either run by local optometrists or by retinal photography, to ensure that expert assessment is made.[1] Standards and quality assurance guidance for the national retinopathy screening programme are available.[3]

Designing the audit

Selection of sample

Look at all patients on the diabetic register.

Prospective or retrospective

The audit has to be retrospective because of the nature of the data.

Collecting the data

- Run a search for the code for retinal screening for all patients on the diabetic register.
- Check the medical records of a sample, e.g. one in ten, to establish that those who should be referred for treatment have been referred to ophthalmologists.

Who will collect the data?

- A member of the primary care team trained in audit searches.
- The health professional lead on diabetes management.

Resources required to complete the audit

- Designated time for the searches.
- The lead clinician needs time to search the computer or written medical records for information about referral.
- Time for all the relevant members of the practice team to meet and discuss the findings and agree the way in which changes will be implemented.

Who will analyse and present the data?

The lead clinician on diabetes management is ideal.

Feeding back and negotiating change

You should look at the changes required with all the team members involved. For example, the audit may indicate:

- the direct referral arrangements are working well for patients who have been screened by the centrally organised programme. No action is needed
- elderly or housebound patients on the diabetes register are not being screened. A protocol is drawn up. A letter, form and list of centres will be sent to the patient who can arrange an appointment with one of the optometrists listed who carry out domiciliary visits. Alternatively, they can make an appointment to attend the acute trust for retinal photography, and transport can be arranged for housebound patients, if necessary. The appointment can be made by a relative or a carer or by the GP practice. Patients will be recalled on an annual basis
- some patients who live in one area of the practice attend an optometrist who is not part of the local scheme. Referral recommendations from this optometrist are sent to the practice, and some appear to have been lost or not acted upon. The practice makes a request to the primary care organisation to include this optometrist in the centrally organised scheme so that referrals can be made direct (as the other optometrists do). Until that can be changed, the secretary agrees to collect all optometrist referral forms to ensure the relevant clinician authorises referral
- some patients who have attended digital retinopathy photography sessions have been recalled to attend a biomicroscopy slit examination, as their results could not be graded. The audit identifies that none of the recalled patients from your practice have attended this centre. The practice nurse contacts these few patients by telephone and finds that the centre is situated in a pedestrianised precinct some distance from any parking or public transport. This information is passed back to the primary care organisation responsible for the commissioning of the retinopathy service.

Influencing changes resulting from the audit

The lead clinician is responsible for monitoring whether the changes agreed are followed through.

Planning to re-audit

Re-audit the referrals in 6 months to ensure the changes have been successful. Re-audit all in 12 months to ensure that the changes regarding housebound patients are working.

References

1 Chambers R, Stead J and Wakley G (2001) *Diabetes Matters in Primary Care.* Radcliffe Medical Press, Oxford.

2 Sharp PF, Olsen J, Strachan F *et al.* (2003) *The Value of Digital Imaging in Diabetic Retinopathy.* NHS Health Technology Assessment, London. www.hta.nhsweb.nhs.uk

3 www.nscretinopathy.org.uk/pages/nsc.asp?ModT=A&Sec=16

Audit template

Transient ischaemic attack and stroke 1: secondary prevention

Select the topic and review the literature

An audit topic should concern an area that has at least one of the following characteristics:

(1) high risk
(2) high volume
(3) causes concern
(4) high cost

Many of the patients on the stroke and transient ischaemic attack (TIA) register will also appear on the registers of other domains of the QOF, such as diabetes, coronary heart disease or hypertension (2). Prevention of further attacks is focused on reducing hypertension (*see* the hypertension template, page 66), cholesterol levels and antiplatelet or anticoagulant therapy (1 and 3).[1] Disability from stroke is likely to increase as the population ages, so preventing further attacks in people who are at high risk because of previous TIAs or minor strokes reduces the cost to individuals and society (4).[2]

Criteria

The QOF states that the practice can show that the percentage of:

Criteria	Maximum threshold (minimum 25%)	Points
Treatment with aspirin/other antiplatelet or an anticoagulant recorded in the notes of patients with a confirmed history of a non-haemorrhagic stroke or history of a TIA	90%	4
Total cholesterol recorded in the previous 15 months	90%	2
Last total cholesterol level 5 mmol/l or less, measured in the previous 15 months	60%	5

Standards

Standards should be:

- realistic
- measurable
- achievable
- agreed

The standards in the QOF will be difficult to meet. It is easy to measure total cholesterol levels but difficult to reduce them. Patients often have indigestion on antiplatelet medication (and stop them) and monitoring of warfarin is difficult in patients, like these, who often have multiple disabilities and illnesses. You might want to start at low levels, e.g. the minimum threshold of 25%. When you repeat the audit, set your standards higher than the last time. Ensure that your registers are as accurate as possible. Record as exemptions refusals, contraindications, adverse reactions and maximal treatment. Look at the levels of therapy and ensure that treatment is maximised to try to reach the target figures or below.

Clinical Evidence reports that the evidence is lacking that antiplatelet agents other than aspirin are effective and that high dose aspirin is no more effective and more likely to cause harm.[3] Most people should be on low dose (75 mg) aspirin, with or without gastroprotective agents such as misoprostol, H_2 inhibitors or proton pump inhibitors.[4]

Designing the audit

Selection of sample

You might want to obtain maximal reward for your efforts by starting with those patients who appear on more than one register, e.g. diabetes, coronary heart disease and left ventricular dysfunction.

Prospective or retrospective

The audit has to be retrospective because of the nature of the data.

Collecting the data

Run a search every six months to establish how near you are to your target.

Who will collect the data?

- A member of the primary care team trained in audit searches.

- A designated health professional looks for the clinical data missing from the computer record and for the reasons.

Resources required to complete the audit

- Patient records kept contemporaneously on a computer system make this audit easy to complete, provided clinicians enter the data under the agreed Read codes.
- Designated time to do the searches.
- The health professional must have designated time to analyse the data and propose the necessary changes.
- Time for all the relevant members of the practice team to meet and discuss the findings and agree the way in which changes will be implemented.

Who will analyse and present the data?

The analysis is likely to involve a health professional looking at clinical or patient reasons for failure to achieve the required levels, and adding exception coding to patient records as necessary.

Feeding back and negotiating change

You should look at the changes required with all the practice team members involved. For example, the audit may indicate:

- lower levels of aspirin use than expected
  - some patients who have to pay prescription charges purchase their own aspirin. Record this at their medication review
  - patients have stopped taking it because of indigestion. Change to alternatives or add a gastroprotective agent (whichever is advised by the prescribing lead as the most cost-effective)
- good recording of the last cholesterol level
- many patients with cholesterol levels above 5 mmol/l. The clinicians agree to increase the statin doses to maximum to try to achieve a cholesterol level of 4 mmol/l or less.

Influencing changes resulting from the audit

The lead clinician is responsible for monitoring whether the changes agreed are followed through. Do not re-audit too soon; these changes will take time to show.

Planning to re-audit

Revise the standards ready for the next round, taking into account the changes that have been agreed. Re-audit after 12 months.

References

1 Wakley G, Chambers R and Ellis S (2004) *Demonstrating Your Competence 3: Cardiovascular and Neurological Conditions.* Radcliffe Publishing, Oxford.

2 Intercollegiate Stroke Working Party (2004) *National Clinical Guidelines for Stroke.* Clinical Effectiveness and Evaluation Unit, Royal College of Physicians, London. www.rcplondon.ac.uk/pubs/books/stroke/stroke_guidelines_2ed.pdf

3 Godlee F (ed.) (2004) *Clinical Evidence Concise.* Issue 11. BMJ Publishing, London. www.clinicalevidence.com

4 Joint Formulary Committee (2004) *British National Formulary.* British Medical Association and Royal Pharmaceutical Society, London. www.bnf.org

Transient ischaemic attack and stroke 2: practice protocol

Select the topic and review the literature

An audit topic should concern an area that has at least one of the following characteristics:

(1) high risk
(2) high volume
(3) causes concern
(4) high cost

After a transient ischaemic attack (TIA), the risk of a stroke within the next month can be as high as one in five, with the highest risk occurring within the first few days (1).[1] Each year over 130 000 people in England and Wales have a stroke (2). A quarter of a million people are living with long-term disability as a result of stroke in the UK (4). TIAs should be treated as vigorously and quickly as acute coronary syndrome. Three main areas of delay in treatment occur (3):

- patients do not understand the urgency of the condition and present late
- the primary care team does not respond with sufficient urgency
- the secondary care system is too poorly resourced to respond quickly.[2]

This audit looks at the performance of the primary care team and identifies areas where improvements might be required.

Criteria

The National Service Framework for Older People for England states that, by April 2004, primary care trusts will ensure that:

- all practices use protocols agreed with local experts to treat and identify patients at risk of stroke
- all GP practices have an agreed protocol for rapid referral for TIA.[3]

The revised *National Clinical Guidelines for Stroke* include recommendations for the management of TIAs (*see* under Standards).[4]

Standards

Standards should be:

- realistic
- measurable
- achievable
- agreed

If you have only just introduced a protocol, your level of achievement will probably be lower than if it has been in place for some time. If you are repeating the audit, set your standards higher than the last time.

Criteria	Example of standard
Patients with a possible diagnosis of TIA, or who have had a stroke with good recovery by the time they are seen, should be referred urgently for investigation as soon as possible within 7 days of the incident	70%
Patients with a possible diagnosis of TIA should be prescribed aspirin (300 mg), or other antiplatelet medication, immediately	90%
Patients with more than one TIA in a week should be investigated in hospital immediately	90%
Patients with a TIA should have a blood pressure check two weeks after the event	80%

Designing the audit

Selection of sample

The numbers involved will not be large, so all patients with a new possible diagnosis of TIA or recovered stroke can be included in the sample. A general practitioner with a list size of 2000 people will see five new people with a TIA or a stroke each year.[5]

Prospective or retrospective

If you instituted the above standards some time in the past, e.g. from April 2004, you could start with a retrospective study of all patients from that date for 12 months. However, as these are new standards, it makes sense to select a date by which you feel everyone should be aware of the criteria, and start a prospective audit of all patients seen from then on for 12 months.

Collecting the data

You need a way of identifying people who have a possible diagnosis *before* confirmation and coding as a TIA or stroke. Agree a method, e.g.:

- a written register
- a database entry into Excel, Epi Info or similar simple statistical package
- a retrievable Read code such as a symptom 'loss of power' (the easiest for audit).

At intervals, e.g. every three months, search the records of the selected sample and record the level of compliance with the standards.

Who will collect the data?

- The responsibility for identifying the patient as being part of the sample rests with the clinician, so all health professionals must be committed to the audit.
- The collection of the data after the patient is registered as part of the sample can be delegated to a member of the primary care team trained in audit searches.

Resources required to complete the audit

- Patient records kept contemporaneously on a computer system make audits much easier to complete, provided clinicians enter the data under the agreed Read codes.
- The audit can be done with a written list of eligible patients and a manual search of paper records, as the numbers involved are small.
- Training and information for clinicians and audit staff are essential for correct audit procedures.
- Designated time to do the searches.
- The lead clinician must have designated time to analyse the data and propose the necessary changes, and may need training in the preparation of simple statistical data or in presentation skills.
- Time for all the relevant members of the practice team to meet and discuss the findings and agree the way in which changes will be implemented.

Who will analyse and present the data?

A health professional lead on stroke prevention and care is ideally situated to analyse and present the data. The lead clinician should also monitor the interim results, be a point of contact for any queries and encourage the rest of the team to continue to identify patients for the sample.

Feeding back and negotiating change

Feed back the results to a meeting of all the relevant members of the practice team and to the primary care organisation. For example:

- the audit may identify a lack of appreciation of the urgency of the condition by reception staff, the district nurses or pharmacists. Involve them in an educational session

- fewer than expected patients are identified as part of the sample. Tackle the awareness of the diagnosis among clinicians in an educational session
- a delay in referral occurs because of lack of available appointments in the rapid access TIA clinic. Feed back this information to the primary care organisation
- the main cause of delay identified is lack of appreciation by patients of the urgency, with many patients presenting later than 7 days after the event. A patient information campaign is planned with leaflets and posters obtained or designed by the health visitor.

Influencing changes resulting from the audit

The lead clinician is responsible for monitoring whether the changes agreed are followed through.

Planning to re-audit

Agree a date for re-audit at the time of the presentation. The practice manager or audit clerk may be responsible for entering this into a timetable of planned audits, so that it does not clash with others.

References

1 Coull AJ, Lovett JK and Rothwell PM (2004) Oxford Vascular Study. Population based study of early risk of stroke after transient ischaemic attack or minor stroke: implications for public education and organisation of services. *British Medical Journal.* **328**: 326–8.

2 Wakley G, Chambers R and Ellis S (2004) *Demonstrating Your Competence 3: Cardiovascular and Neurological Conditions.* Radcliffe Publishing, Oxford.

3 Philp I and Platt D (co-chairmen External Reference Group) (2001) *National Service Framework for Older People.* Department of Health, London.

4 www.rcplondon.ac.uk/pubs/books/stroke/stroke_conciseguide_2ed.pdf

5 www.prodigy.nhs.uk/guidance.asp?gt=TIA%20-%20not%20in%20AF

Audit template
Hypothyroidism 1: monitoring

Select the topic and review the literature

> An audit topic should concern an area that has at least one of the following characteristics:
>
> (1) high risk
> (2) high volume
> (3) causes concern
> (4) high cost

Hypothyroidism occurs in around 4 in 1000 women on average, rising to 8 in 1000 people over 70 years old (2). Mean incidence is 3.5 per 1000 for women and 0.6 per 1000 for men. In a practice of approximately 9000 patients, there will be around 500 to 600 patients taking levothyroxine, giving a prevalence of approximately 6%.[1]

Women are six times more likely to suffer from hypothyroidism than men. Higher rates of myocardial infarction and atherosclerosis occur in hypothyroidism (1). Depression and memory impairment are associated with hypothyroidism.[1,2] It is easy to miss the gradual onset of hypothyroidism, and symptoms and signs take a long time to become evident after discontinuation of medication (3).

Criteria

The QOF states that the practice can show the percentage of:

Criteria	Maximum threshold (minimum 25%)	Points
Patients on the hypothyroidism register with a thyroid function test in the last 15 months	90%	6

You should also ensure that action is taken following the thyroid function test and that a date for the next test is set (*see* below).

Standards

Standards should be:

- realistic
- measurable
- achievable
- agreed

With any long-term condition, the risks of failure to take the prescribed medication are considerable, especially as the effects are subtle in the early stages of under-replacement. People miss tablets or fail to take them for a considerable period before clinical effects of hypothyroidism recur. If blood levels of thyroid stimulating hormone are in the therapeutic range then annual review is sufficient, but, if not, more frequent tests and adjustment of medication are required.[2] You might add these criteria (*see* table below) to this audit of the QOF (*see* above).

Criteria	*Standard*
Patients on the hypothyroidism register have a record that their dose of levothyroxine has been reviewed following the most recent thyroid function test	90%
Patients on the hypothyroidism register have a record of the date for the next thyroid function test	90%

Designing the audit

Selection of sample

Look at all the patients taking levothyroxine.

Prospective or retrospective

The audit has to be retrospective because of the nature of the data.

Collecting the data

- Search for the data listed above for patients on the hypothyroidism register.
- A trained member of the clerical staff will have to search the free text entries on computer or the written medical notes for the data that is missing.

Who will collect the data?

- A member of the primary care team trained in audit searches.
- The trained member of the clerical staff.

Resources required to complete the audit

- Designated time to do the searches.
- The health professionals responsible for the reviews of patients with hypo-thyroidism have training and enough time to enter the data into the template.
- The trained clerical staff member needs designated time to search the computer free text or written medical records for missing data.
- Time for all the relevant members of the practice team to meet and discuss the findings and agree the way in which changes will be implemented.

Who will analyse and present the data?

The practice manager or trained clerical staff member might take the responsibility.

Feeding back and negotiating change

You should look at the changes required with all the practice team members involved. For example, the audit may indicate:

- a lack of training in the use of the computer and lack of time for the health professionals involved, so that information is not recorded in a retrievable form. It is agreed that the trained clerical staff member will train two others. All thyroid function results will be annotated by the clinicians with the recommended dosage and date of the next test, and put in a file. The trained clerical staff will record the information on the computer. The information will be added to the right-hand side of the repeat prescription, so that the patient is informed and reminded
- difficulty establishing whether patients are being advised about dosage changes and the next date for their thyroid function test. *See* above for changes agreed
- the proportion of patients attending for thyroid function tests is only 45%. An information leaflet about the importance of regular testing is obtained and attached to each prescription over the next 12 months.[3,4]

Influencing changes resulting from the audit

The lead clinician and/or practice manager are responsible for monitoring whether the changes agreed are followed through. They may need to support training or education, e.g. in correct management, coding or in patient information and the queries arising from that process.

Planning to re-audit

Have a timetable of planned audits, so that this regular audit does not clash with others. Revise the standards ready for the next round, taking into account the changes that have been agreed.

References

1 Chambers R, Wakley G and Pullan A (2004) *Demonstrating Your Competence 4: Respiratory Disease, Mental Health, Diabetes and Dermatology.* Radcliffe Publishing, Oxford.

2 Godlee F (ed.) (2004) *Clinical Evidence Concise.* Issue 11. BMJ Publishing Group, London. www.clinicalevidence.com

3 www.prodigy.nhs.uk

4 www.btf-thyroid.org

Audit template
Hypothyroidism 2: patients at risk

Select the topic and review the literature

An audit topic should concern an area that has at least one of the following characteristics:

(1) high risk
(2) high volume
(3) causes concern
(4) high cost

Patients are at risk following treatment or resolution of an overactive thyroid (1). Primary hypothyroidism occurs after destruction of the thyroid gland because of an autoimmune state (i.e. chronic autoimmune thyroiditis) or medical intervention such as surgery, radioiodine or radiation treatment. It may occur as a side-effect from drugs such as amiodarone or lithium. Secondary hypothyroidism occurs after damage to the pituitary gland or hypothalamus.[1] Patients who are treated with radioiodine or thyroid surgery should be placed on a practice disease register and have their thyroid function tested annually.[2,3] Fifty per cent will become hypothyroid over time and require prescribed levothyroxine (3). Signs and symptoms of hypothyroidism are subtle and gradual, so that disability and loss of function may be present for some time if screening is not performed (4).

Criteria

Good practice suggests that:

Criteria	Standard
Patients who are treated for thyrotoxicosis should be placed on a practice disease register and have their thyroid function tested annually	90%

Standards

Standards should be:

- realistic
- measurable
- achievable
- agreed

Aim to try and follow up everyone with a history of treatment for an overactive thyroid. You should be able to give sufficient information about the subtle symptoms of an underactive thyroid to convince most people that annual screening is worthwhile. A blood test showing results of a thyroid stimulating hormone (TSH) level over 12 mU/l and a low serum thyroxine (T4 less than 60 nmol/l) confirms the diagnosis.

Designing the audit

Selection of sample

Look at all the patients who have had treatment for thyrotoxicosis.

Prospective or retrospective

The audit has to be retrospective because of the nature of the data.

Collecting the data

- Search for all patients with a diagnosis of thyrotoxicosis or treatment with carbimazole or propylthiouracil.
- Search for evidence that those people compiled by the above search have had a thyroid function test in the last 15 months.
- A trained member of the clerical staff will have to search the free text entries on computer or the written medical notes for the data that are missing.

Who will collect the data?

- A member of the primary care team trained in audit searches.
- The trained member of the clerical staff.

Resources required to complete the audit

- Designated time to do the searches.

- Training and enough time for the health professionals responsible for the reviews of patients with hypothyroidism to enter the data into the template.
- The trained clerical staff member needs designated time to search the computer free text or written medical records for missing data.
- Time for all the relevant members of the practice team to meet and discuss the findings and agree the way in which changes will be implemented.

Who will analyse and present the data?

The health professional with an interest in thyroid disease might take the responsibility.

Feeding back and negotiating change

You should look at the changes required with all the practice team members involved. For example, the audit may indicate:

- more patients than expected are identified from the recently summarised and computerised records and very few have had a recent thyroid function test. The practice team agrees that:
  - the practice secretary will print out an information leaflet about the risks of hypothyroidism after treatment for thyroxicosis.[4] She will mail this out with a covering letter to all those identified to recall them for blood tests during April, May and June
  - the health visitor offers to put on a display of information about thyroid disease in the waiting room
  - extra appointment slots are allocated for the expected blood tests
- the senior partner is sure that some patients are missing from the register found by searching, but cannot immediately identify any missing names
  - the health visitor says she will add two posters to her display asking patients who have had treatment to fill in a file card (kept in boxes below the posters) with their name, address and date of birth and hand it to the receptionist
  - the audit clerk will add any patients not previously identified to the register
- the practice team identify that they will have to add patients to the register proactively. The practice secretary and the coding clerks will all identify patients proactively from referral and discharge data, to add to the list.

Influencing changes resulting from the audit

The lead clinician and/or audit clerk are responsible for monitoring whether the changes agreed are followed through.

Planning to re-audit

Repeat the audit after the last call for blood tests have been completed, e.g. in August to determine if the changes have been successful.

References

1 Chambers R, Wakley G and Pullan A (2004) *Demonstrating Your Competence 4: Respiratory Disease, Mental Health, Diabetes and Dermatology*. Radcliffe Publishing, Oxford.

2 National Prescribing Centre (2001) Management of Thyroid Disease. MeRec Bulletin. **13(3)**: 9–12. www.npc.co.uk/MeReC_Bulletins/2001Volumes/pdfs/vol12no3.pdf

3 Vanderpump MP, Ahlquist JAO, Franklyn J *et al.* (1996) Consensus statement for good practice and audit measures in the management of hypothyroidism and hyperthyroidism. Research Unit of the Royal College of Physicians, Endocrinology and Diabetes Committee of the Royal College of Physicians and the Society for Endocrinology. *British Medical Journal.* **313**: 539–44.

4 www.netdoctor.co.uk/diseases/facts/hyperthyroidism.htm

Audit template

Cancer 1: register

Select the topic and review the literature

> An audit topic should concern an area that has at least one of the following characteristics:
>
> (1) high risk
> (2) high volume
> (3) causes concern
> (4) high cost

An ageing population means that larger numbers of patients will develop cancer (1 and 2). Cancer care is a government priority. Although patients with cancer are mainly managed in secondary care, primary care plays an important role in co-ordination of care and support.[1,2] Co-ordination can improve care by preventing duplication of effort, improving liaison between the various individuals and organisations involved, and acting as advocates for patients when required (3 and 4).

Criteria

The QOF states that the practice can show it has a:

Criteria	Maximum threshold (minimum 25%)	Points
Register of patients with cancer, excluding non-melanotic skin cancers, diagnosed after April 2003	Within expected prevalence	6

In a small practice, the incidence of cancer over a couple of years may be very different from the population incidence due to chance alone. Practices with a higher proportion of older patients will have a higher incidence.

Standards

Standards should be:

- realistic
- measurable
- achievable
- agreed

Obtain the expected incidence per year for cancers in your area from the primary care organisation's public health lead. You should aim to record all the patients as the diagnosis is confirmed. Eventually, your cumulative incidence each year should correspond sufficiently well with the public health estimates, unless your practice population is very different from the average, e.g. includes mainly mothers and children in the vicinity of a naval base. One of the major difficulties in meeting the requirements of the QOF register is that a search carried out at the end of the year will exclude patients who have died during the year.

Pharmacists become aware of significant presenting symptoms and refer patients to their GP promptly, especially if their symptoms have persisted for several weeks. Patients requesting repeated supplies of laxatives, anti-diarrhoeal drugs, mouth ulcer preparations or antacids should trigger the need for counselling. This should be handled sensitively, to avoid causing anxiety for the patient, but the importance of seeking prompt medical advice should be emphasised. Some areas have put in place a GP referral document, agreed locally, listing symptoms that should be referred and a referral letter from the pharmacist to the GP detailing the symptoms described and history of medicines used. You might arrange a meeting to put this into place to increase the early identification of cancers.

Cancer care is also covered elsewhere in the QOF, e.g. significant event analysis, smoking cessation.

Designing the audit

Selection of sample

Search for entries in the relevant codes since 1 April 2003.

Prospective or retrospective

The audit has to be retrospective because of the nature of the data.

Collecting the data

- Compare your results with the expected incidence over the relevant period, e.g. 24 months.

- Involve all primary care staff, including district nurses, receptionists, etc in collecting information about patients who have a diagnosis of cancer on index cards.

Who will collect the data?

A member of the primary care team trained in audit searches.

Resources required to complete the audit

- Designated time to do the searches.
- All staff need to have a supply of index cards on which to record patient details. Use a template on the card so that people are encouraged to complete it as fully as possible, e.g. name, address, date of birth, diagnosis and consultant if known.
- All the relevant members of the practice team need to meet and discuss the findings and agree the way in which changes will be implemented.

Who will analyse and present the data?

The lead clinician on cancer management in your practice is ideal.

Feeding back and negotiating change

You should look at the changes required with all the practice team members involved. For example, the audit may indicate:

- poor recording of the diagnosis on the computer. It is agreed to:
  - print out a list of suitable codes, laminated and placed in each consulting and treatment room. Look at guidelines for the relevant cancers[3]
  - ask doctors to highlight the diagnosis on hospital letters and the data entry clerks to check whether the diagnosis has been entered on the computer record and tick the diagnosis in green pen
- anecdotal evidence of delays before letters are received from secondary care following the diagnosis of cancer. The secretary agrees to keep a list of those referred with suspected cancer and record their progress in secondary care in tabular form. If this delay is confirmed, representations will be made to the medical director at the trust and to the primary care organisations.

Influencing changes resulting from the audit

The lead clinician is responsible for monitoring whether the changes agreed are followed through.

Planning to re-audit

Annual audit will be sufficient if data are being recorded consistently on the computer. If not, schedule them more frequently to monitor the changes.

References

1 Wakley G, Chambers R and Gerada C (2004) *Demonstrating Your Competence 5: Substance Abuse, Palliative Care, Musculoskeletal Conditions, Prescribing Practice*. Radcliffe Publishing, Oxford.

2 Wakley G and Chambers R (eds) (2005) *Chronic Disease Management in Primary Care: quality and outcomes*. Radcliffe Publishing, Oxford.

3 http://rms.nelh.nhs.uk/guidelinesFinder

Audit template

Cancer 2: reviews

Select the topic and review the literature

> An audit topic should concern an area that has at least one of the following characteristics:
>
> (1) high risk
> (2) high volume
> (3) causes concern
> (4) high cost

You need to decide as a practice team how cancer care reviews will be organised as no evidence-based criteria exist. The patient journey can be divided into:

- initial consultation with the GP and referral
- hospital outpatient clinics and investigations
- any inpatient episode
- oncology treatment
- discharge: community and palliative care.

Cancer care reviews should take place at any stage after diagnosis to ensure that care is as seamless as possible, so focus audit alongside.[1] Involve as many members of the patient care team as required, remembering that delivering cancer care is very much a team activity. There will be many people under review at any one time (2), requiring complicated multidisciplinary action (3) and using a large amount of NHS resources (3).

Criteria

The QOF states that the practice can show that:

Criteria	Maximum threshold (minimum 25%)	Points
Patients with cancer diagnosed after 1 April 2003 have a review recorded within six months of confirmed diagnosis	90%	6

The review should include an assessment of support needs and a review of co-ordination with and between different aspects of secondary care. Management should be based on national and local guidance.[2]

You might want to look at patient-held records to facilitate the interchange of information. It is often difficult to motivate the many individuals involved to duplicate their records by entering information into a patient-held record as well as their own records, but it is a very useful way of making sure that everyone knows what is being done and who has said what to whom.[3]

Standards

Standards should be:

- realistic
- measurable
- achievable
- agreed

The main difficulty is in retrieving the information, as the various practice team members may record their activity in many different ways. Start with a low standard such as 25% and analyse your findings to see where the difficulties lie.

Make sure that you discuss with patients and carers what information they feel that they need.[4]

Designing the audit

Selection of sample

The QOF suggests that the practice searches for those patients added to the cancer register between six and 12 months ago who have a code for 'cancer diagnosis discussed', e.g. 8BAV.00. Unless all clinicians have agreed to use this code, it may be preferable to also look through the written or computer records of all patients added to the cancer register between six and 12 months ago.

Prospective or retrospective

The audit has to be retrospective because of the nature of the data.

Collecting the data

Compare your results of the searches for the code and the examination of the records.

Who will collect the data?

A member of the primary care team trained in audit searches. A clinician may need to be involved in the examination of consultation records, to make a decision about when a review of patient needs has been completed.

Resources required to complete the audit

- Designated time to do the searches.
- All the relevant members of the practice team need to meet and discuss the findings and agree the way in which changes will be implemented.

Who will analyse and present the data?

The lead clinician on cancer management in your practice is ideal.

Feeding back and negotiating change

You should look at the changes required with all the practice team members involved. For example, the audit may indicate:

- poor recording of the review on the computer. It is agreed that:
  - in future, all clinicians will use the agreed Read code when undertaking a review
- difficulties in establishing what the review has included. A structured template linked to the code will be used to record the review and management plans. A copy will be printed out for the patient.

Influencing changes resulting from the audit

The lead clinician is responsible for monitoring whether the changes agreed are followed through.

Planning to re-audit

Check in 3–6 months to see if the right Read codes are being used and the template is being completed. Annual audit will be sufficient if data are being recorded consistently on the computer. If not, schedule them more frequently to monitor the changes.

References

1   Wakley G and Chambers R (eds) (2005) *Chronic Disease Management in Primary Care: quality and outcomes.* Radcliffe Publishing, Oxford.
2   www.nelh.nhs.uk

3 NHS Modernisation Agency: Cancer Services Collaborative. *Patient-held Records Toolkit.* www.modern.nhs.uk/cancer/5628/7050/Patient-Held%20Records3.pdf

4 Chambers R, Drinkwater C and Boath E (2003) *Involving Patients and the Public: how to do it better* (2e). Radcliffe Medical Press, Oxford.

Audit template

Mental health 1: lithium medication

Select the topic and review the literature

An audit topic should concern an area that has at least one of the following characteristics:

(1) high risk
(2) high volume
(3) causes concern
(4) high cost

Bipolar disorder is a recurring illness and one of the leading causes of worldwide disability (2). It is especially disabling in the age groups 15 to 44 years when people are usually at their most productive (1 and 4). The lifetime prevalence of suicide in people with bipolar disorder is around 2%, which is 15 times greater than expected (2).[1]

Criteria

The QOF states that the practice can show the percentage of:

Criteria	Maximum threshold (minimum 25%)	Points
Patients on lithium therapy with a record of lithium levels checked in the last six months	90%	3
Patients on lithium therapy with a record of lithium levels in the therapeutic range in the last six months	70%	5
Patients on lithium therapy with a record of serum creatinine and thyroid stimulating hormone in the past 15 months	90%	3
Additional criteria not part of the QOF: Patients with a lithium information card	90%	Not applicable

Standards

Standards should be:

- realistic
- measurable
- achievable
- agreed

The therapeutic range for lithium is usually 0.6–1.0 mmol/l. If the range acceptable locally is different, you will need to inform the primary care organisation. Levels below this therapeutic range are acceptable for some individuals, depending on the clinical condition.[2]

Patients on lithium who are literate should have a lithium card, obtainable from pharmacies, that tells patients how to take lithium preparations, what to do if a dose is missed and what side-effects to expect. It also explains why regular blood tests are important and warns about drug interactions and the effects of illnesses on lithium levels.[3] Set your standard at 90%. Arrange a meeting so that practices and pharmacies can decide how to check that patients have a lithium card.

Designing the audit

Selection of sample

Look at all the patients taking lithium.

Prospective or retrospective

The audit has to be retrospective because of the nature of the data.

Collecting the data

- Search for all patients on lithium, and for the relevant data recorded in their medical records (listed above).
- Examine the written or computer records for the criteria listed above if they are missing from coded information.
- Ask every patient collecting a prescription for lithium if they have a lithium information card.

Who will collect the data?

- A member of the primary care team trained in audit searches.
- The health professional lead on mental health management.
- The pharmacists and their assistants.

Resources required to complete the audit

- Designated time to do the searches.
- The lead clinician needs time to search the computer free text or written medical records for any missing data.
- A meeting with the local pharmacists who will explain to their staff the necessity for checking if patients taking lithium have information cards.
- Additional lithium cards for anyone who needs one.
- Time for all the relevant members of the team to meet and discuss the findings and agree the way in which changes will be implemented.

Who will analyse and present the data?

The lead clinician on mental health management in your practice is ideal.

Feeding back and negotiating change

You should look at the changes required with all the team members involved. For example, the audit may indicate:

- missing data because the blood is taken at a lithium clinic and results not copied to the practice. The lead professional discusses the problem with the lithium clinic. It is agreed that the results of investigations will be copied to the practice by the laboratory, but the clinic will retain the responsibility for contacting the patient to alter the dose, or take other action, if required
- many patients have no lithium information card. Non-judgemental discussion at the lithium clinic reveals that this was because they did not realise that this was important information and threw them away or did not read them. The pharmacists and pharmacy assistants agree to add a short verbal explanation of the purpose of the cards and to continue enquiring, when patients collect a prescription, whether patients have a copy.

Influencing changes resulting from the audit

The lead clinician is responsible for monitoring whether the changes agreed are followed through.

Planning to re-audit

Re-audit in 12 months to establish if the changes agreed are effective.

References

1 Godlee F (ed.) (2004) *Clinical Evidence Concise* Issue 11. BMJ Publishing Group, London. www.clinicalevidence.com

2 Chambers R, Wakley G and Pullan A (2004) *Demonstrating Your Competence 4: Respiratory Disease, Mental Health, Diabetes and Dermatology.* Radcliffe Publishing, Oxford.

3 Joint Formulary Committee (2004) *British National Formulary.* British Medical Association and Royal Pharmaceutical Society of Great Britain, London. www.bnf.org

Audit template

Mental health 2: medication for depression

Select the topic and review the literature

An audit topic should concern an area that has at least one of the following characteristics:

(1) high risk
(2) high volume
(3) causes concern
(4) high cost

The prevalence of major depression is between 5% and 10% of the people seen in primary care settings (2). Two to three times as many people have depressive symptoms of a lesser severity. Depressive disorders are the fourth most common cause of disability worldwide (4).[1] Antidepressant drugs account for 7% of UK primary care drug expenditure, and untreated depressed patients use two to three times the annual medical services compared to their non-depressed counterparts (4).[2] Antidepressant medication is effective when used properly, but many patients discontinue medication too soon or do not take them because of fears of addiction or side-effects (3).[2] Depression is a stronger predictor of serious cardiac disease during the year following cardiac catheterisation than smoking, severity of coronary artery disease and diminished left ventricular ejection fraction (1).[2]

Criteria

You should have a protocol for managing depression in line with the *National Service Framework for Mental Health.*[3] You might include in your protocol the items in Table AT2.

Consult the current advice from the Committee on Safety of Medicines about the use of antidepressants.[4]

Table AT2: Criteria for a protocol for management of depression[2]

	Yes	No

Patients are:

- given an explanation of depression
- offered an antidepressant and/or non-drug therapy and support
- reviewed after 2–3 weeks on an antidepressant to assess thoughts of self-harm and side-effects
- given an adjusted dose or alternative antidepressant, or continued for at least six months
- reviewed regularly for six months

If it is the first episode, the dosage is gradually reduced

If more than three episodes have occurred in 5 years, long-term therapy is discussed

Standards

> Standards should be:
> - realistic
> - measurable
> - achievable
> - agreed

You might want to agree to start with a standard of 70% for adherence to the protocol. The protocol should be agreed by all clinical staff and have been in use for at least six months before the audit.

Designing the audit
Selection of sample

You might choose to look at all first presentations of depression in a period of 12 months. In view of the number of people you are likely to identify, it might be preferable to choose a sampling method, e.g. 1 in 10, to select smaller numbers.

Prospective or retrospective

The audit has to be retrospective because of the nature of the data.

Collecting the data

- Search for and list the (sample of) patients with a diagnosis of depression.
- Examine the written or computer records for the criteria listed above.

Who will collect the data?

- A member of the primary care team trained in audit searches.
- The health professional interested in mental health management.

Resources required to complete the audit

- Designated time to do the searches.
- The health professional needs protected time to search the computer free text or written medical records for the information required by the protocol.
- Time for all the relevant members of the practice team to meet and discuss the findings and agree the way in which changes will be implemented.

Who will analyse and present the data?

The health professional interested in mental health management is ideal.

Feeding back and negotiating change

You should look at the changes required with all the practice team members involved. For example, the audit may indicate:

- the first consultation is generally well recorded in accordance with the protocol. No action is needed
- many patients started on antidepressant medication do not return after 2–3 weeks or for regular review but re-attend in a crisis. The practice team agrees that they must improve the information given to the patients about the rationale and the risks and benefits of treatment.[2] The practice manager orders a supply of leaflets on depression[5]
- poor recording of the assessment of the likelihood of self-harm at the first review consultation. This is important information for the prevention of harm and modification of management. It may prove essential in the event of a complaint. All staff involved in monitoring the patient's progress agree to record these data at review.

Influencing changes resulting from the audit

The health professional interested in mental health management is responsible for monitoring whether the changes agreed are followed through. He or she may need to support training or education, e.g. in correct management or in patient information and the queries arising from that process.

Planning to re-audit

Re-audit in 12 months to establish if the changes agreed are effective.

References

1 Godlee F (ed.) (2004) *Clinical Evidence Concise* Issue 11. BMJ Publishing Group, London. www.clinicalevidence.com

2 Chambers R, Wakley G and Pullan A (2004) *Demonstrating Your Competence 4: Respiratory Disease, Mental Health, Diabetes and Dermatology.* Radcliffe Publishing, Oxford.

3 National Health Service Executive (2000) *National Service Framework for Mental Health.* Department of Health, London. Full version: www.dh.gov.uk/assetRoot/04/07/72/09/04077209.pdf and executive summary on: www.dh.gov.uk/assetRoot/04/01/45/01/04014501.pdf

4 Committee on Safety of Medicines (last updated 8 April 2004) *Selective Serotonin Reuptake Inhibitors (SSRIs): overview of regulatory status and CSM advice relating to major depressive disorder (MDD) in children and adolescents including a summary of available safety and efficacy data.* medicines.mhra.gov.uk/ourwork/monitorsafequalmed/safetymessages/ssrioverview_101203.htm

5 Leaflets available from the Royal College of Psychiatrists: www.rcpsych.ac.uk/info/dep.htm

Audit template
Medicines management 1: repeat prescriptions

Select the topic and review the literature

An audit topic should concern an area that has at least one of the following characteristics:

(1) high risk
(2) high volume
(3) causes concern
(4) high cost

Around 1.8 million prescriptions are written by GPs in England every day (2 and 4).[1] Defence societies report that there are about 200 claims involving medicines made against GPs each year and the potential for harm from incorrect prescriptions is large (1). One estimate of the frequency of preventable adverse drug events gave it as nearly 2% of all patients admitted to hospital, while another study of GP prescription errors averted by watchful pharmacists put the frequency of those errors as one in 10 000 (3).[1] Accuracy is essential, but a rapid turn around is required to ensure that medication is available to be taken.[2]

Criteria

The QOF states:

- *Medicines 4.1 Practice guidance*: practices should provide a reasonably fast service for their repeat prescriptions. Details of how the practice's system works should be contained in the practice leaflet
- *Medicines 4.2 Written evidence*: the practice leaflet or policy is available
- *Medicines 4.3 Assessment visit*: the receptionists are questioned on the policy
- *Medicines 4.4 Assessors' guidance*: the assessors should check that the system for issuing repeat prescriptions can be described by the receptionists and should observe it in action.

An audit will demonstrate the policy in action.

Criteria	Points
The number of hours from requesting a prescription to availability for collection by the patient is 72 h or less (excluding weekends and bank/local holidays)	3
The number of hours from requesting a prescription to availability for collection by the patient is 48 h or less (excluding weekends and bank/local holidays)	6

Standards

Standards should be:

- realistic
- measurable
- achievable
- agreed

Your audit standard is the same as that in the patient leaflet, e.g. 95% of prescriptions are available within 48 h from the request.

Designing the audit

Selection of sample

It will be difficult and cumbersome to select a random sample of prescriptions for audit. Although less accurate, a sample of all the prescriptions for a defined four-week period would give sufficient information for analysis of any problems. The period can be selected randomly (*see* below).

Prospective or retrospective

The audit has to be retrospective because of the nature of the data.

Collecting the data

Make it simple to operate at the frontline so that it can easily be repeated at intervals. Conceal when it is being monitored or staff may make extra effort temporarily.

- All prescriptions taken out of the collection box, received in the post, or handed in at the desk are stamped with the date (e.g. blue for a.m. and green for p.m.).

- The prescription is processed in the normal way, but request slips are routinely kept with the prescription (not shredded when the prescription is printed).
- If a problem arises, this is written on the request slip.
- When ready to be collected (or posted or sent to the pharmacy), the request slip is date stamped again in the relevant colour.
- The request slips are passed routinely to the audit clerk who shreds all but those being audited at intervals.

Who will collect the data?

Any member of the primary care team trained in audit.

Resources required to complete the audit

- Designated time for the audit searches.
- Time for all the relevant members of the practice team to meet and discuss the findings and agree the way in which changes will be implemented.

Who will analyse and present the data?

Record the proportion falling within the stated time. Record the stated reasons for difficulties and whether this caused delay beyond the stated time. Circulate the results and then discuss them at a joint clinical and administrative meeting.

Feeding back and negotiating change

Look at the changes required with all the practice team members involved. The audit may indicate that delay occurs because of:

- patient factors: requested too early, requested item is not on the repeat list, unclear what items are needed, the review date has been exceeded
- staff factors: no-one available to process requests in the afternoon, queries to doctors are lost in the pile of mail awaiting attention.

Influencing changes resulting from the audit

- The team agrees that receptionists will practise some role-play with the practice nurse on how best to explain the repeat prescription system to patients who have made inappropriate requests. The practice manager arranges a meeting with local pharmacists to discuss how they can help.
- The prescription requests containing queries for doctors are put in bright coloured folders on top of the pile of post awaiting attention, and the doctors agree to attend to those speedily.
- The practice manager suggests changing to a system that he has seen in other practices. Prescriptions could be ordered by telephone with direct checking by the prescription clerk with the patient as to the availability of the repeat medication in

the computer medical record. He is asked to look at the resource implications of this change.
- The practice manager agrees to look at staffing levels and activities in the afternoon, to see if a receptionist can be released to deal with prescription requests, so that some prescriptions could be ready for signing before morning surgeries the following day. The practice manager or senior receptionist will be responsible for monitoring whether the changes agreed are being implemented and are working.

Planning to re-audit

It is agreed that the practice manager or senior receptionist will arrange a re-audit within a specified time at dates of their choosing and report back to the practice team. If the system is working well, no formal discussion will be needed until other changes are suggested.

References

1 Wakley G, Chambers R and Gerada C (2005) *Demonstrating Your Competence 5: Substance Abuse, Palliative Care, Musculoskeletal Conditions, Prescribing Practice*. Radcliffe Publishing, Oxford.
2 Audit Commission (1994) *A Prescription for Improvement*. HMSO, London.

Medicines management 2: continuation of treatment

Select the topic and review the literature

> An audit topic should concern an area that has at least one of the following characteristics:
>
> (1) high risk
> (2) high volume
> (3) causes concern
> (4) high cost

In secondary prevention of cardiovascular disease, treatment with medication is a high priority[1] to reduce risk (1), involves many patients (2), and is expensive for the health service (4). Start by comparing the rates of continuation of medication in this group of patients – those discharged from hospital after a cardiovascular event such as a myocardial infarction.[2] Around 20% of patients studied were not taking their medication within six months of being discharged from hospital.[3,4] You could carry out a similar exercise looking at the use of other medication in patients who have asthma, chronic obstructive pulmonary disease (COPD) or diabetes.

Criteria

You will only be able to measure whether patients are regularly ordering the prescribed medication. You will not be able to establish if they are stockpiling the packets in a cupboard at home!

You should be able to demonstrate that at least some of the secondary prevention measures recommended by research studies are being successfully implemented.[5]

Standards

> Standards should be:
>
> • realistic
> • measurable
> • achievable
> • agreed

Set your standards by consultation with your colleagues. You might want to make an aspirational target following the actual results from the study quoted above. These are given in the criteria list below. When you repeat the audit, you will want to set your standards higher than the last time.

Criteria	Standard (e.g. as found in the American study[4])
At six months after discharge from hospital, patients who were discharged on these drugs have ordered sufficient to provide them with the daily dose*:	
aspirin	92%
beta-blocker	88%
ACE inhibitor or angiotensin converting drug	80%
statin	87%

*Unless there are specific contraindications to that therapy[2]

Designing the audit

Selection of sample

The annual rate for a first or recurrent coronary event per 100 000 population aged less than 65 years, in 1994–1995, was 273 for men and 66 for women, after age adjustment to a standard world population.[6] Sample all the patients discharged from hospital on these medications in the last 24 or 36 months to obtain a reasonable number to analyse. Some will not have been discharged on those medications because of contraindications or other medical conditions, so you will probably have about 26 per 10 000 patient list per year.

Prospective or retrospective

The audit has to be retrospective because of the nature of the data.

Collecting the data

- Search for patients discharged from hospital with a myocardial infarction within the dates specified.
- Record those with full compliance in the first six months after discharge from hospital.
- A health professional looks at the 'non-compliant' patients to find any reasons why the medication has not been requested. For example, an adverse reaction to the drug, aspirin being purchased by a patient not exempt from prescription charges, or other contraindications have developed since the first prescription.

Who will collect the data?

• A member of the primary care team trained in audit searches.
• A designated health professional looks at the clinical data for the patients who are 'non-compliant'.

Resources required to complete the audit

• The audit can be done with a written list of eligible patients and a search of computerised repeat medication records, as the numbers involved are small.
• Designated time for audit searches.
• The health professional must have protected time to analyse the data and propose the necessary changes.
• Time for all relevant members of the practice team to meet and discuss the findings and agree the way in which changes will be implemented.

Who will analyse and present the data?

Normally a GP or nurse practitioner will lead on cardiovascular prevention and care. The health professional involved in looking at recorded reasons for 'non-compliance' may be the best person to analyse and present the data after discussion with the lead clinician. The analysis is likely to involve looking at other reasons for 'non-compliance' and an understanding of the difference between compliance and concordance.[7,8]

Feeding back and negotiating change

Look at the changes required with all the practice team members involved. For example, the audit may indicate:

• a lack of appreciation by patients of the importance of the medication in preventing further attacks. You may want to find, or write, an information leaflet with reinforcement of the advice by the health professionals when medication is reviewed
• resistance by patients to adopting a 'sick role' requiring medication including denial of ill-health or ignoring the risks. The practice must be prepared to let some patients take an informed decision not to take medication, and record their wishes
• exclusion of patients from potentially preventive medication by inappropriate application of contraindications, e.g. stopping aspirin because of indigestion instead of adding a gastroprotection.

Influencing changes resulting from the audit

The lead clinician is responsible for monitoring whether the changes agreed are followed through. He or she may need to support training or education, e.g. in repeat prescription management, or in patient information, and the queries arising from that process.

Planning to re-audit

Re-audit as part of planned programme of audits.

References

1 Joint Formulary Committee (2004) *British National Formulary.* British Medical Association and Royal Pharmaceutical Society, London. www.bnf.org

2 Godlee F (ed.) (2004) *Clinical Evidence Concise* Issue *11.* BMJ Publishing Group, London. www.clinicalevidence.com

3 www.jr2.ox.ac.uk/bandolier/booth/Pharmacy/ebtadher.html

4 Eagle KA, Kline-Rogers E, Goodman SG *et al.* (2004) Adherence to evidence-based therapies after discharge for acute coronary syndromes: an ongoing prospective, observational study. *American Journal of Medicine.* **117**: 73–81.

5 Dovey S, Hicks N, Lancaster T *et al.* (1998) Secondary prevention of coronary heart disease: how completely are research findings adopted in practice. *European Journal of General Practice.* **4**: 6–10.

6 Volmink JA, Newton JN, Hicks NR *et al.* (1998) on behalf of the OXMIS Study Group. Coronary event and case fatality rates in an English population: results of the Oxford Myocardial Infarction Incidence Study. *Heart.* **79**: 40–4.

7 www.ub.uio.no/umn/farm/pbl/artikler/hypertens5.pdf

8 Marinker M, Blenkinsopp A, Bond C *et al.* (eds) (1997) *From Compliance To Concordance: achieving shared goals in medicine taking.* Royal Pharmaceutical Society of Great Britain, London.

Audit template
Patient information needs 1: telephone consultations

Select the topic and review the literature

An audit topic should concern an area that has at least one of the following characteristics:

(1) high risk
(2) high volume
(3) causes concern
(4) high cost

Good Medical Practice for General Practitioners states that the excellent GP 'has a system for receiving or returning phone calls from patients' and that the unacceptable GP 'provides no opportunity for patients to talk to a doctor or a nurse on the phone'(1).[1]

Some practices have specific times to speak to a clinician and others make arrangements for the clinician to phone the patient back. This information can be advertised to patients through the practice leaflet, notices in the practice, slips given to patients when being asked to phone back for a result, the tear-off side of a prescription, the practice newsletter, etc.

The Department of Health reported in 2002 that 21% of patients had said that 'on at least one occasion in the last 12 months the surgery receptionist had made it difficult for them to see or talk to the doctor' (3).[2] The great majority of respondents reported that surgery receptionists were helpful (2). The proportion of respondents who said that they could not always – or even on most occasions – get through to the surgery on the telephone at the first attempt had increased since the last survey – from 39% to 42%.[2]

Criteria

The QOF states that the practice can show:

Criteria for patient access for advice or information	Possible standard	Points
The practice has arrangements for patients to speak to GPs and nurses on the telephone during the working day	A written policy	1
Patients are able to obtain the information that they require from a relevant member of the practice staff after one or two attempts at contact	90%	Good practice
Patients are aware of the arrangements for contacting the relevant member of the practice staff	70%	Good practice
Patients are able to access a receptionist via telephone and face to face in the practice, for at least 45 hours over 5 days, Monday to Friday, except where agreed with the primary care organisation	For the hours stated	1.5

Standards

Standards should be:

- realistic
- measurable
- achievable
- agreed

The reception staff can answer many of the queries that patients pose. You should have guidelines about what information the reception staff can give, e.g. the results of investigations, or how to access particular health provision. A practice nurse, suitably trained, may be able to give advice about the management of minor illnesses or the need to make an appointment for medical conditions.

Designated time for answering telephone queries helps to meet patient need. All this information should be advertised to patients so that they feel able to use the system efficiently. Possible standards are given in the chart above.

Designing the audit

Selection of sample

The reception staff note down the identification of all telephone callers over a four-week period. The annual patient survey is used to provide data about people who might not have used the telephone or were unable to get through.

Prospective or retrospective

The audit has to be both prospective (for the patients who telephone) and retrospective (from the patient survey).

Collecting the data

- Data on any difficulties in getting through to the surgery are collected from the patient satisfaction survey.
- A record is completed for each patient who phoned for information:

Patient identifier   *Recorded answers*

Has the patient phoned before about this query?

Who answered the query?

Was the patient satisfied with the information?

Was the query passed to another practice team member
and who was this?

Has the patient any suggestions how the practice could
improve the service?

Who will collect the data?

- Every member of the practice team answering queries.
- The practice manager collating the answers to the patient satisfaction survey.

Resources required to complete the audit

- Extra time for the reception staff answering the phone for queries. Some other reception duties are reduced during the survey period to allow for this extra time.
- Designated time for the doctors, practice nurses, health visitors, midwives, etc so that they are available to answer queries relevant to their expertise.

Who will analyse and present the data?

The practice manager might take the responsibility.

Feeding back and negotiating change

You should look at the changes required with all the practice team members involved. For example, the audit may indicate:

- patients were not aware of the designated times for telephone encounters and many did not find them convenient, especially if they had to ring again. Several patients commented that they would prefer email contact as being more convenient. The practice made plans to enable secure email posting and answering of queries to add to the already implemented repeat prescription service. Details about the present and new arrangements would be advertised by messages on the repeat prescription tear-off side, posters and in the practice leaflet that was being re-issued
- the reception staff often found that patients were not happy about the amount of information that the receptionists could give about the results of investigations. There was insufficient information written by the clinician who had reviewed the result. The receptionists found saying 'the results are normal' often made people frustrated. The wording for normal results was changed to 'no abnormal results have been found, please make an appointment if your symptoms continue'. Clinicians agreed to try and write what they would like the patient to be told about any investigation
- the midwives and health visitors found that they could not guarantee to be at the surgery at the advertised times to answer the phone. They agreed that, for them, a better system was for the receptionists to pass the patients' details to their mobile phones and they would phone the patient back as soon as they could. They did not feel comfortable with using email to answer queries, so were not included in the proposed new facility.

Influencing changes resulting from the audit

The practice manager is responsible for monitoring whether the changes agreed are followed through.

Planning to re-audit

Having tackled a specific problem, you may find that the regular patient satisfaction survey meets your needs for auditing whether the changes have met the patient need.

References

1 Royal College of General Practitioners and General Practitioners Committee (2001) *Good Medical Practice for General Practitioners*. Royal College of General Practitioners/General Practitioners Committee, London.

2 www.dh.gov.uk/PublicationsAndStatistics/PublishedSurvey/ NationalSurveyOfNHSPatients/GPSurvey19992002/GPSurveyArticle/fs/ en?CONTENT_ID=4001356&chk=McLwIb

Patient information needs 2: informed choice

Select the topic and review the literature

> An audit topic should concern an area that has at least one of the following characteristics:
>
> (1) high risk
> (2) high volume
> (3) causes concern
> (4) high cost

The Healthcare Commission is encouraging patients to take a more active role in managing their health or illness (1).[1] It suggests that, among other question, patients should ask:

- do I get the right information and explanations at the right time?
- am I able to make real choices about my healthcare?

You can assess whether you are meeting the needs of patients in your practice for information and what problems arise when trying to meet those needs. Poor information leads to poor compliance and complaints (1, 3 and 4).

Criteria

Criteria for information for patients	Possible standard	Points
Information about common conditions is readily available for patients to take away with them	90%	Good practice
Information about less common conditions can be found and supplied to patients on request	70%	Good practice
The practice supports smokers in stopping smoking by a strategy that includes providing literature and offering appropriate therapy	Practice protocol exists	2

Standards

Standards should be:

- realistic
- measurable
- achievable
- agreed

The practice team does not need to write its own smoking cessation strategy but can adopt a local or national protocol.[2] The provision of dedicated smoking cessation services remains the responsibility of the primary care organisation.

Similarly, you can use information about guidelines for treatment and general information about common conditions obtained from any source – provided someone in the practice team has approved the content or the source. For example, you might use Prodigy patients' information leaflets (PILs), or the patient information website.[3,4] The standards you might achieve are listed in the criteria above.

Designing the audit

Selection of sample

All requests for information are collected over a four-week period and the availability of information to meet that request noted.

Prospective or retrospective

The audit has to be prospective.

Collecting the data

All members of the practice team and the local pharmacists agree to take part. Each person has a record sheet on which to record a patient identifier, the information required and how the request was dealt with, e.g. a leaflet found, printed out, handwritten information, etc.

Who will collect the data?

- Every member of the team answering queries.
- The practice manager and one receptionist with a special responsibility for information supply, collate the record sheets.

Resources required to complete the audit

- Extra time for the reception staff answering the phone for queries.
- Leaflets are catalogued alphabetically or obtained by printing out.
- A good supply of smoking cessation information is on display in the waiting area and available in each consulting room. The receptionist with a special responsibility for information supply keeps the stock renewed.
- The local pharmacists agree to stock *Family Doctor* booklets and some free leaflets.[5]

Who will analyse and present the data?

The practice manager might take the responsibility.

Feeding back and negotiating change

You should look at the changes required with all the practice team members involved. For example, the audit may indicate:

- a lack of information about specific problems, especially obesity and special dietary considerations for illnesses. The receptionist responsible will contact the dietitian to ask her advice about suitable leaflets
- some staff have problems locating information on the computer and printing it out. The practice manager undertakes to provide extra training
- it was noticed that some of the leaflets in the filing cabinets are out of date, or contain promotional material by the company supplying them. They are removed from the supply. The receptionist responsible for leaflets, the health visitor and the registrar will look for alternatives
- there was no known source of information for some less common conditions. The practice manager arranged for one of the librarians to come and give a tutorial on how to search for reliable information on the internet
- smoking cessation information is always very well stocked and staff have found it easy to supply. The receptionist responsible is congratulated
- the pharmacists comment that patients think that the *Family Doctor* booklets should be provided free and that few sales have been achieved. They also found that many of the leaflets that they stocked were promotional, as pharmaceutical firms had supplied them free of charge. They have decided not to continue stocking either, but will liaise with the practice team about suitable non-promotional leaflets.

Influencing changes resulting from the audit

The practice manager and responsible receptionists agree to monitor whether the changes agreed are followed through.

Planning to re-audit

Repeat the audit in about 12 months to establish whether the changes have been successful.

References

1 www.healthcarecommission.org.uk/assetRoot/04/00/02/21/04000221.pdf

2 www.nice.org.uk/pdf/NiceNRT39GUIDANCE.pdf

3 www.prodigy.nhs.uk/PILs/index.asp

4 www.patient.co.uk/pils.asp

5 www.bma.org.uk/ap.nsf/Content/bmabooksonhealth

Audit template
Back pain 1: diagnostic triage

Select the topic and review the literature

> An audit topic should concern an area that has at least one of the following characteristics:
>
> (1) high risk
> (2) high volume
> (3) causes concern
> (4) high cost

Morbidity studies in general practice show that the consultation rate for back pain has risen in the past 10 years (2). Forty per cent of adults responding to the Office for National Statistics Omnibus Survey in Great Britain in 1998 said they had suffered from back pain lasting for more than one day in the previous 12 months (3).[1] The prevalence of persistent back pain increased with age: around one in three men and one in four of women aged 65 years and over suffered for the whole year with back pain, compared with around one in 12 men and women aged between 25 and 44 years (1).[1] Back pain is also very expensive (4) (*see* Back pain audit 2: referral, page 153).

Criteria

In order to check whether everyone is acting as a team, agree local guidelines and audit whether everyone is following them. Arrange a meeting with pharmacists, GPs, osteopaths, chiropractors and physiotherapists to agree what the local treatment guidelines and referral procedures should be. Local guidelines should be based on the national guidelines, e.g. those published by the Royal College of General Practitioners.[2] Look first at the initial assessment by the professional of first contact. This may be a pharmacist, nurse practitioner, GP, etc. Criteria for diagnostic triage of back pain are given in Table AT3.

Table AT3: Table of criteria for a protocol for diagnostic triage of back pain[2]

	Yes	No

The following questions have established that simple backache is likely:

- patient between 20 and 55 years of age
- site of pain is lumbosacral, buttocks and thighs
- pain varies with physical activity and time
- the patient is well otherwise

	Yes	*No*

**Nerve root pain has not been present for more than
4 weeks and is resolving with time. Nerve root pain includes**:

- unilateral leg pain worse than low back pain
- radiation to foot or toes
- numbness or paraesthesia in the same distribution
- nerve irritation signs – reduced straight leg raising,
  which reproduces leg pain
- motor, sensory or reflex change – limited to one nerve root

Questions have excluded 'red flags', i.e.:

- age of onset less than 20 or more than 55 years
- violent trauma, e.g. fall from height, road traffic accident
- constant, progressive, non-mechanical pain
- thoracic pain
- past medical history of carcinoma, systemic steroids
- drug abuse, HIV
- systematically unwell
- weight loss
- persisting severe restriction of lumbar flexion
- widespread neurology
- structural deformity

**Questions have excluded widespread neurological disorder
(cauda equina syndrome):**

- difficulty with micturition
- loss of anal sphincter tone or faecal incontinence
- saddle anaesthesia about the anus, perineum or genitals
- widespread or progressive motor weakness in the legs or gait
- disturbance

Positive messages for simple backache have been given:

- backache is very common
- activity is helpful, too much rest is not
- advise patients to stay as active as possible and to continue
- normal daily activities
- advise patients to increase their physical activities progressively
- over a few days or weeks
- if a patient is working, then advice to stay at work or return to
- work as soon as possible is probably beneficial
- X-rays are not indicated
- no referral to other practitioner necessary within 4–6 weeks if
  improving
- analgesics to be taken at regular intervals, not as required
- any contraindications to NSAIDs established
- any additional comments from the professional seeing the patient

NSAID: non-steroidal anti-inflammatory drug

Look at *Clinical Evidence* for guidance on types of treatment for acute back pain.[3]

Standards

Standards should be:

- realistic
- measurable
- achievable
- agreed

You might want to agree to start with a standard of 70% for adherence to the protocol. The protocol should be agreed by all participants and have been in use for at least three months before the audit to ensure everyone is used to it.

Designing the audit

Selection of sample

You might choose to look at all new presentations of back pain in a four-week period.

Prospective or retrospective

The audit has to be prospective as the patients present.

Collecting the data

After each patient has been seen, fill in the check sheet to establish if you have followed the protocol.

Who will collect the data?

All involved in the audit.

Resources required to complete the audit

- Designated time to fill in the check sheet after seeing the patient.
- A nominated or volunteer professional to collect and collate the data.
- Time for all involved to meet, discuss the findings and agree the way in which changes will be implemented.

Who will analyse and present the data?

The volunteer or nominated professional who collated the check sheets is ideal.

Feeding back and negotiating change

You should look at the changes required with all involved. For example, the audit may indicate:

- many patients have difficulty retaining the information given verbally and present again, or to other professionals for the same advice. Non-promotional leaflets and useful websites[4,5] are obtained for distribution to patients
- some professionals found that it was too time consuming to go through all the questions and often suggested that patients should return to see them or another professional after a week if the pain has not gone. Discussion concluded that it was a better use of time, as well as being safer, to do the assessment properly the first time the patient presented. Several people pointed out that inadequate assessment and advice perpetuated the psychosocial ideas about back pain associated with poor resolution.

Influencing changes resulting from the audit

Those more experienced in managing back pain offered to support by phone or email those professionals who needed to make the most changes.

Planning to re-audit

Re-audit in 12 months to establish if the changes agreed are effective.

References

1 Office for National Statistics (2004) *Social Trends. Census 2001.* www.statistics.gov.uk/STATBASE/xsdataset.asp?vlnk=674

2 Foord-Kelcey G (ed.) (2004) *Guidelines Vol 24.* Medendium Group Publishing Ltd, Berkhamsted, Herts. http://www.eguidelines.co.uk

3 Godlee F (ed.) (2004) *Clinical Evidence Concise* Issue 11. BMJ Publishing Group, London. www.clinicalevidence.com

4 www.bbc.co.uk/health/conditions/back_pain/

5 www.backcare.org.uk/index2.php

Audit template

Back pain 2: referral

Select the topic and review the literature

An audit topic should concern an area that has at least one of the following characteristics:

(1) high risk
(2) high volume
(3) causes concern
(4) high cost

Back pain is common and causes much disability (1 and 2). At least 5 million adults consult their GP annually concerning back pain. This leads to costs in primary care of £141 million. NHS physiotherapy costs are estimated at £151 million. Ten per cent of those complaining of back pain visited a complementary practitioner (osteopath, chiropractor, acupuncturist). NHS hospital costs (outpatients, accident department, daycare and inpatients) are estimated at £512 million.[1] Work-related costs are also high as back pain is the leading cause of disability with 1.1 million people affected in the UK (4).[2]

Criteria

Local guidelines should be based on the national guidelines, e.g. those published by the Royal College of General Practitioners.[3] Look to see if referrals made are helpful and not just wasting time for a colleague. Any audit of this nature should be multidisciplinary, with each professional looking at his or her own practice and sharing the results, so that everyone involved learns from the process. Criteria for referral of back pain are given in Table AT4.

Table AT4:   Table of criteria for a protocol for referral criteria for back pain

	Yes	*No*

Nerve root pain has been present for more than 4 weeks and is not resolving with time. Nerve root pain includes:

- unilateral leg pain worse than low back pain
- radiation to foot or toes
- numbness or paraesthesia in the same distribution
- nerve irritation signs – reduced straight leg raising, which
- reproduces leg pain
- motor, sensory or reflex change – limited to one nerve root

Questions have revealed one or more 'red flags', i.e.:

- age of onset less than 20 or more than 55 years
- violent trauma, e.g. fall from height, road traffic accident
- constant, progressive, non-mechanical pain
- thoracic pain
- past medical history of carcinoma, systemic steroids
- drug abuse, HIV
- systematically unwell
- weight loss
- persisting severe restriction of lumbar flexion
- widespread neurology
- structural deformity

Or questions have revealed widespread neurological disorder (cauda equina syndrome):

- difficulty with micturition
- loss of anal sphincter tone or faecal incontinence
- saddle anaesthesia about the anus, perineum or genitals
- widespread or progressive motor weakness in the legs or gait disturbance
- referred for manipulative treatment within the first six weeks as
- patient needs additional help with pain relief or is failing to return to normal activities
- referred for reactivation/rehabilitation as patient has not returned to ordinary activities and work within six weeks
- space for any comments from the professional seeing the patient

Look at *Clinical Evidence* for guidance on types of treatment for acute and chronic back pain.[4]

Standards

Standards should be:
• realistic • measurable • achievable • agreed

You might want to agree to start with a standard of 70% for adherence to the protocol. The protocol should be agreed by all participants and have been in use for at least a few months before the audit.

Designing the audit

Selection of sample

You might choose to look at all presentations of back pain in a 12-week period where referral took place.

Prospective or retrospective

The audit has to be prospective as the patients present.

Collecting the data

After each patient has been seen, fill in the check sheet to establish if you have followed the protocol.

Who will collect the data?

All involved in the audit.

Resources required to complete the audit

• Designated time to fill in the check sheet after seeing the patient.
• A nominated or volunteer professional to collect and collate the data.
• Time for all involved to meet and discuss the findings and agree the way in which changes will be implemented.

Who will analyse and present the data?

The nominated or volunteer professional who collated the check sheets is ideal.

Feeding back and negotiating change

You should look at the changes required with all involved. For example, the audit may indicate:

- some professionals found that pressure from patients, rather than clinical assessment, prompted a referral. It was agreed that advice should be reiterated but that some flexibility in referral was necessary according to the degree of urgency or anxiety felt by the patient. Patient leaflets and other information were felt to be helpful in reinforcing the advice given[5,6]
- it was difficult to discover whether referrals were appropriate, as patients were often lost to follow-up once referred. It was agreed to organise another meeting with the physiotherapists, osteopaths and chiropractors in the area to discuss referrals and establish if there was any way feedback could be improved.

Influencing changes resulting from the audit

Those more experienced in managing back pain offered to support by phone or email those professionals who needed to make the most changes.

Planning to re-audit

Re-audit in 12 months to establish if the changes agreed are effective.

References

1   Palmer KT, Walsh K, Bendall H *et al.* (2000) Back pain in Britain: comparison of two prevalence surveys at an interval of two years. *British Medical Journal.* **320**: 1577–8.

2   Klaber Moffett J, Richardson G, Sheldon TA and Maynard A (1995) *Back Pain: its management and cost to society.* Centre for Health Economics, University of York.

3   Foord-Kelcey G (ed.) (2004) *Guidelines Vol 24.* Medendium Group Publishing Ltd, Berkhamsted, Herts. www.eguidelines.co.uk

4   Godlee F (ed.) (2004) *Clinical Evidence Concise* Issue 11. BMJ Publishing Group, London. www.clinicalevidence.com

5   www.bbc.co.uk/health/conditions

6   www.backcare.org.uk/index2.php

Audit template

Patient safety 1: sterilisation of instruments

Select the topic and review the literature

An audit topic should concern an area that has at least one of the following characteristics:

(1) high risk
(2) high volume
(3) causes concern
(4) high cost

Sterilising instruments in the general practice or dental environment to a high standard is essential to reduce the risk of cross-infection (1). Minor surgical procedures are often undertaken in primary care increasing the risk (2). Any surgical instrument used on a patient becomes a potential source of infection to another patient and to anyone handling the instrument (3). To minimise the risk, each instrument must be cleaned and sterilised as soon as possible.

HTM 2030 is the NHS Standard governing the washing and disinfection of surgical and dental instruments. HTM 2010 is the NHS Standard for instrument sterilisation. Together HTM 2030 and HTM 2010 establish the benchmark for safe, effective surgical instrument decontamination.[1]

Criteria

You should have a protocol for sterilisation of instruments. High risk medical devices penetrate skin or mucous membrane, and enter the vascular system or sterile spaces. Intermediate risk items come into contact with intact mucous membranes or may be contaminated with particularly virulent or readily transmissible organisms. They require high level treatment to remove vegetative bacteria. Low risk items are those that either contact only intact skin or do not come into contact with the patients.[2] Criteria for sterilisation of instruments are given in Table AT5.

Table AT5:   Example criteria for a protocol for sterilisation of instruments in high or moderate risk use

	Yes	No
Sterile and dirty instruments are clearly segregated		
All instruments are transported in appropriate rigid containers		
All contaminated instruments are washed thoroughly before sterilisation*		
Staff handling contaminated instruments are trained to minimise the risk of infection to themselves		
Protective clothing, e.g. gloves (and aprons and eye/face protection if washing instruments) is provided to staff handling contaminated instruments		
All washers, sterilisers, ultrasonic baths, etc are cleaned regularly in line with accepted good practices regarding method and regularity for the particular make and model*		
A record of the routine regular maintenance and calibration of decontamination equipment is kept*		
Potential risk or actual harm from cross-infection is examined as a significant event		

* Not relevant if you send the instruments to a central sterile service department

Standards

Standards should be:
- realistic
- measurable
- achievable
- agreed

You might agree to have a standard of 100% for adherence to the protocol, as it is so important.

Designing the audit
Selection of sample

A check of the criteria should be made by an unscheduled visit by the 'infection control nurse' from the primary care organisation.

Prospective or retrospective

The audit has to look at what happens on the day of the visit and also retrospectively at the records kept.

Collecting the data

The infection control nurse:

- observes the staff procedures when dealing with contaminated instruments
- examines the records and any significant event analysis or potential or actual risk from cross-infection kept by the designated manager for prevention of cross-infection.

Who will collect the data?

- The infection control nurse.
- The designated manager responsible for cross-infection control for the practice, e.g. a senior nurse.

Resources required to complete the audit

- Some scheduled work for that day may have to be postponed to allow time for the detailed inspection.
- The designated manager for prevention of cross-infection needs time to supervise the procedures and keep records.
- Training needs for staff must be identified and met.
- Time for all the relevant members of the practice team to meet and discuss the findings and agree the way in which changes will be implemented.

Who will analyse and present the data?

The designated manager for prevention of cross-infection is ideal.

Feeding back and negotiating change

You should look at the changes required with all the practice team members involved. For example, the audit may indicate:

- the infection control nurse passes on her congratulations to the practice team for generally high standards
- contaminated instruments are being moved from one room to another in a gloved hand, potentially exposing others to infection. The practice will purchase a supply of rigid boxes that can also be sterilised
- some instruments are difficult to clean adequately before sterilisation. The manager will investigate the possibility of replacing these with disposable instruments

- few episodes of potential risk have been recorded. The infection control nurse feels that under-recording is likely from her experience of other practices. She encourages staff to report any events for non-judgemental examination.

Influencing changes resulting from the audit

The designated practice lead for prevention of cross-infection will review the training needs for staff especially in the area of reporting risks of cross-infection.

Planning to re-audit

Another unscheduled visit will be made.

References

1   www.decontamination.nhsestates.gov.uk

2   Royal College of Nursing (2004) *Good Practice in Infection Control*. Royal College of Nursing, London. www.rcn.org.uk/publications/pdf/goodpracticeinfectioncontrol.pdf

Audit template
Patient safety 2: resuscitation

Select the topic and review the literature

> An audit topic should concern an area that has at least one of the following characteristics:
>
> (1) high risk
> (2) high volume
> (3) causes concern
> (4) high cost

Cardiopulmonary collapse occurs relatively rarely, but the practice team should have up-to-date skills to deal with an emergency. Regular practical skills-based training sessions are required, as it is known that these skills diminish after a relatively short time (1 and 3). This training may be available from a variety of providers including your local accident and emergency department, BASICS, the primary care organisation or out-of-hours co-operative, Red Cross, St John's Ambulance or equivalent. It may be sufficient for one individual in the team to attend for external training and then cascade this within the team.[1] Automatic defibrillator equipment is now available at a reasonable cost (4).

Criteria

The timescale for basic life support training within the QOF has been set pragmatically at 18 months, although many general medical practices offer training for staff on a more frequent basis.

Pharmacists, dental practitioners, physiotherapists and other professionals allied to medicine should consider adhering to similar criteria and auditing their standards.

All members of the primary care team who have contact with patients should be trained and equipped, to a level appropriate for their expected role, to resuscitate patients who suffer cardiopulmonary arrest in the community. The minimum standard should be proficiency in basic life support. Consider training for everyone so that they have the skills to react appropriately. For example, if you ever have the situation where a doctor runs late when only the cleaners are present, you might want to offer training to the cleaners as well. The majority of the team should be capable (with appropriate training) of using an automated external defibrillator (AED).[1] Criteria for provision of life support are given in Table AT6.

Table AT6:   Criteria for provision of immediate life support

	Yes	*No*
There is a record of all practice-employed clinical staff having attended training/updating in basic life support skills in the preceding 18 months	4 points	
All clinical staff have similarly had their basic life support skills updated and recorded for their appraisal documentation		
The location of equipment and emergency drugs is clearly indicated on the premises and known to staff		
A protocol for calling for assistance and making a 999 call exists and is known to staff		
A named member of staff, and a deputy in his/her absence, is responsible for the regular inspection and maintenance of emergency equipment		

Standards

> Standards should be:
> - realistic
> - measurable
> - achievable
> - agreed

In this important area, you might want to set a standard for 95% of staff to have received basic life support training within the previous 18 months (to allow for new members of staff to have time to receive training).

Designing the audit

Selection of sample

All staff should be included.

Prospective or retrospective

A snapshot audit looks at skills at the time of the training session. Carry out a review of emergency equipment and knowledge on the same occasion.

Collecting the data

- Arrange a training/updating session in paid time for all staff, inviting anyone who works with patients on the premises to attend.
- Each person at the training session should have an opportunity to practise with a resuscitation trainer so that they know they have the requisite skills.
- The trainer will review knowledge about the protocol and equipment. The emergency equipment should also be inspected.

Who will collect the data?

- The trainer will assess the skills, the knowledge and the state of the equipment.
- The practice manager should record the results.

Resources required to complete the audit

- Protected time for the instruction session.
- Time for all the relevant members of the practice team to meet and discuss the findings and agree the way in which changes will be implemented.

Who will analyse and present the data?

The practice manager is ideal.

Feeding back and negotiating change

You should look at the changes required with all the practice team members involved. For example, the audit may indicate:

- a good level of skills in basic life support by all staff. No other action required
- all drugs are in date and clearly labelled. Equipment is in good condition and suitable for the purpose. The individual responsible is congratulated
- poor knowledge of where the emergency equipment is kept. New laminated notices are placed in each room and all new staff have information about this location included in their induction training
- the oxygen cylinder is large and heavy and could not easily be moved by some of the smaller staff members to where a patient has collapsed. The practice manager will investigate how to obtain a smaller lighter cylinder
- no automatic defibrillator machine is available. No investment in this item had been made because of the cost and the urban location of the practice (ambulance assistance is rapid). The practice team concludes that this is no longer acceptable and the practice manager will look at the cost of providing an automatic defibrillator machine.

Influencing changes resulting from the audit

The practice manager is responsible for monitoring whether the changes agreed are followed through.

Planning to re-audit

Re-audit in 12 months to establish if the changes agreed are effective.

Reference

1   www.resus.org.uk/pages/cpatpc.htm

Index